THE
HIPUS®
REVOLUTION

THE
HIPUS®
REVOLUTION

How Smarter Healthcare IT
Can Save Doctors—and Their Patients

MARK SORENSEN, MD

Advantage | Books

Published by Advantage Books, Charleston, South Carolina.
An imprint of Advantage Media.

ADVANTAGE is a registered trademark, and the Advantage colophon is a trademark of Advantage Media Group, Inc.

Printed in the United States of America.

10 9 8 7 6 5 4 3 2 1

ISBN: 979-8-89188-281-2 (Paperback)
ISBN: 979-8-89188-282-9 (eBook)

Library of Congress Control Number: 2025910352

Cover design by Matthew Morse.
Layout design by Megan Elger.

This publication is designed to provide accurate and authoritative information in regard to the subject matter covered. It is sold with the understanding that the publisher is not engaged in rendering legal, accounting, or other professional services. If legal advice or other expert assistance is required, the services of a competent professional person should be sought.

Advantage Books is an imprint of Advantage Media Group. Advantage Media helps busy entrepreneurs, CEOs, and leaders write and publish a book to grow their business and become the authority in their field. Advantage authors comprise an exclusive community of industry professionals, idea-makers, and thought leaders. For more information go to **advantagemedia.com**.

Dedicated to my family, the greatest blessing in my life.

CONTENTS

PREFACE

WHILE DESIGNING AND PREPARING to implement the HIPUS® system, I encountered radically different responses to this project from healthcare pioneers and nonphysicians (patients) compared with doctors.

A half dozen healthcare pioneers, who have led the way into other uncharted waters, strongly endorsed or expressed great interest in the project.

With few exceptions, nonphysician responses ranged from positive to extremely positive. These individuals asked good questions, clearly understood the need for the HIPUS® system, and very much wanted doctors to use it.

Physician responses were the polar opposite. The vast majority couldn't or wouldn't even talk about it. While working on this project and doing locum tenens (as needed) work in numerous emergency departments, I also found that doctor fear of and resistance to use of such IT is the underlying cause of physician burnout. In fact, such fear helped produce and now sustains burnout.

Implementing the HIPUS® system has so far been impossible for two reasons:

- Doing so isn't possible without physician support and participation.

- A relatively small number of nonphysicians know about the system, and those who do fear alienating doctors by demanding or requesting implementation of the HIPUS® system.

I published this book hoping to remove these barriers by helping more doctors and non-physicians understand the need for such IT, giving nonphysicians a safe and effective way to express their desire for doctor use of it, and prompting physicians to reexamine their resistance to use.

My book coach specializes in helping doctors write books that are easily understood by nonphysicians. We collaborated over several months to achieve that objective. I hope nonphysician readers will find that our efforts were successful. Understanding how the system works will let readers better advocate for its implementation.

The HIPUS® system (pronounced like "hippus" and short for hippocampus, the brain's memory center) is designed *not* to supersede physician memory but to augment that memory and make it more useful.

Use of colors to convey the significance of the presence (specificity) or absence (sensitivity) of findings (signs, symptoms, test results) in ruling in or out diseases is the foundation of the HIPUS® system.

The meanings of the primary (main) and secondary colors are presented in the following images. Secondary colors add to or modify the meanings of the primary colors. When using the system, the secondary color meanings can be quickly accessed or reviewed by tapping on the symbols.

While reading this book and viewing examples of how the system works, you can return to these images and review the meanings.

Primary (main) colors

Purple if present **rule or help rule out**

Green if present **are diagnostic**

Orange and yellow findings are listed in decreasing order of sensitivity. Orange findings always or almost always occur--yellow, less often. Therefore:

Orange if *absent* **rule or help rule out** if present **help rule in**

Yellow if absent don't help much if present **add support to orange**

Secondary colors

Purple, orange, yellow and green are similar to primary colors

X	absence rules out
Xp	absence rules out for all practical purposes
X	absence helps rule out
X	absence doesn't help rule out

●	presence rules out
○	presence helps rule out
●	presence makes very likely
○	presence makes more likely

Blue and brown are the other secondary colors

●	presence warrants further investigation
○	presence is consistent with, but occurs more often with other diseases

INTRODUCTION

IF YOU'RE A PATIENT affected by physician burnout, you're not alone. Several studies and surveys conducted since 2013 have found that about half of all physicians in the US and elsewhere are burned out to the point of compromising care.[1, 2, 3, 4, 5]

The American Medical Association (AMA) defines burnout as a long-term stress reaction, which can include the following:

- emotional exhaustion

- depersonalization (i.e., lack of empathy for or negative attitudes toward patients)

- a feeling of decreased personal achievement[6]

Burnout is a condition that affects all specialists in all practice settings.

In a 2022 Medscape survey, burned-out physicians reported being more easily exasperated with patients, less motivated to take careful patient notes, more likely to express frustration in front of patients, and more likely to make errors.[7]

While working on the HIPUS® project in Philadelphia and doing locum tenens work in emergency departments (EDs) throughout the northeastern region of the US, I found that burnout compromised my care much more than any other factor, including fatigue.

At one point, I had been working on the HIPUS® project when it was at a critical and stressful juncture and had been without much sleep for three days. Before leaving for an ED stint, I was so tired, I hired a cabdriver to take me to Pittsburgh and paid for his flight back to Philly. During that five-hour trip, I was still so wound up I couldn't sleep. In that state, I drove myself from Pittsburgh to Ripley, West Virginia—about 200 miles. After arriving that night, I had to begin my first shift immediately. Needless to say, I was unusually fatigued.

Shortly after my shift began, a nurse said to me: "This child has a fever and purple spots on his skin. What does that mean?" Those findings in a child are usually the only initial signs of meningococcal meningitis, a bacterial infection of the brain, spinal cord, and surrounding membranes. If not treated quickly and very aggressively, it causes death or permanent brain damage. At that point, alarm displaced my fatigue. While consulting with a pediatric infectious disease specialist in Charleston, West Virginia, I performed a spinal tap (inserting a needle into the spinal canal and removing a small amount of spinal fluid), tested the fluid—which confirmed the diagnosis—administered antibiotics and steroids intravenously, and then waited for a special transport team to take the child to Charleston for more advanced treatment than the hospital in Ripley could provide. Children with meningococcal meningitis are so fragile, special transportation is critical. While we were waiting, the patient's condition initially deteriorated but, about thirty minutes before the transport team arrived, began to improve as the antibiotics and steroids kicked in. That specialist later informed me the patient fully recovered without complications. After the transport team left with the patient, my fatigue returned with a vengeance. Fortunately, I had an hour to crash before the next patient arrived.

Unlike fatigue, which didn't compromise my care, burnout did so in a serious way. Several years later, while working at the same hospital and experiencing symptoms of burnout, I cared for an elderly female patient who presented with vague complaints. While working on the HIPUS® project, I studied heart attack and its various symptoms far more than any other disease. After first compiling and organizing information covering heart attack symptoms, I updated the compilation several times over ten years. I therefore certainly should have recalled that elderly patients—especially females with heart attacks—can present with any number of complaints other than chest pain, including vague symptoms. Instead, I was irritated by the patient, assumed she was there because of anxiety/depression or just wanted some attention, and didn't examine her electrocardiogram (ECG) carefully enough. Worse still, I expressed my irritation in front of her and her daughter. The ED director later informed me that the patient returned the next day with similar complaints and her ECG indicated a heart attack. She was successfully treated for it, to my relief. The outcome could have been much worse.

I learned from that experience but eventually quit practicing medicine for two reasons. My response to being repeatedly traumatized and demoralized by the working conditions described in chapter 1 had become unmanageable. I had withdrawn from my family and friends and needed to recover from related drug use. I also realized that the use of much better IT is the only real solution to burnout. I therefore wanted to work full time to develop and implement this much-needed IT.

In fact, use of better IT is the only solution to three interrelated problems, which are seriously harming not only doctors and patients but also everyone else in my country:

- widespread physician burnout

- uneven care quality (adherence to evidence)

- out-of-control cost

This book describes these problems in the United States and explains how use of better IT can effectively address them.

The IT described can help solve the same or similar problems in other nations.

The Institute of Medicine (IOM), now known as the National Academy of Medicine, was established in 1970 as an advisor to the US Congress by the National Academy of Sciences. IOM reports to Congress, published between 2000 and 2013, call for fully integrated use of patient *and care* data to address all three.[8, 9, 10]

I and others are fully prepared to build IT permitting such data use and incorporate it into preexisting electronic health record (EHR) systems.

Chapters one and two discuss physician burnout and show how use of color-assisted, Bayesian-like analysis (CBA) can address that problem.

Chapters three and four are not for everyone. I recommend reading or *not* reading either depending on your interest in the topic and/or related expertise. Chapter three explains the need for CBA to optimize use of AI or machine learning products and let physicians fully interact with those products. Chapter four shows how use of CBA can greatly improve diagnosis-related doctor-nurse collaboration.

Chapters five and six explain the need to improve care quality and reduce costs and show how use of CBA can do so.

While preparing to implement the HIPUS® system, I found that the main barrier to doing so is doctor fear of needed change. Chapter 7 explains what I found to be the cause of such fear and why most doctors can't or won't talk about it. It also describes the radically different responses to this project by healthcare pioneers and nonphysicians versus doctors and how doctor response actually helped produce, and now maintains, burnout. Finally, it explains why physicians needn't fear such change. In fact, needed change will let them lead the way toward solving those three huge problems, secure their rightful place at the center of healthcare, and enjoy more respect, autonomy, and job satisfaction.

Chapter 8 explains why persuading a US emergency medicine physician organization to implement this new IT is the quickest, surest, and most direct way to propel needed change and describes what you can do as a doctor or nonphysician living in the US or elsewhere to help accomplish that task.

CHAPTER 1

Burnout—The Problem

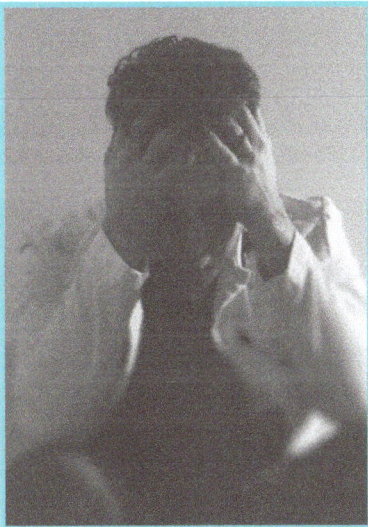

SEVERAL STUDIES AND SURVEYS conducted since 2013 have found that about half of all physicians in the US and elsewhere are burned out.[11, 12, 13, 14, 15] The reasons reported by different specialists are actually quite similar, as are related problems, including withdrawal from family and friends, substance abuse, depression, and suicide. The following focuses on burnout among my colleagues in emergency medicine (EM), which is fairly representative of the problem generally. Methods used to solve the problem in emergency departments (EDs) can be modified for use elsewhere.

Burnout Is Especially Problematic Among Emergency Physicians

In a 2017 Medscape survey, 51 percent of all US physicians and 59 percent of ED physicians reported burnout.[16] Despite efforts to solve the problem via resiliency training, better work–

life balance, peer support, and other such methods, a 2022 Medscape survey found that 47 percent and 60 percent, respectively, were still burned out.[17]

The reasons most often cited by all physicians were

- excessive electronic health record (EHR) tasks (60 percent),

- lack of respect from administrators, colleagues, or staff (39 percent),

- long hours at (or after) work (34 percent), and

- lack of autonomy (32 percent).

Only 12 percent cited pandemic-related reasons.

This chapter first explains the need for use of better IT to address lack of respect and autonomy by letting physicians more easily acquire and demonstrate diagnostic expertise and clearly establish and preserve standard of care—defined as care that is evidence-based, accepted by experts, and widely provided. It then explains the need for improved technology to address excessive EHR tasks and related long working hours by letting doctors document and report care with greater ease and speed.

Such IT is especially needed by emergency physicians.

Physicians Need Better IT to More Easily Acquire and Demonstrate Diagnostic Expertise

While working on the HIPUS® project and doing locum tenens ED work at twenty-six different US hospitals from Massachusetts to Kentucky, I found that lack of respect and autonomy were almost always related to doctors not having a good way to acquire and demonstrate diagnostic expertise.

Dr. Mark Grader, who pioneered efforts to improve diagnosis, once told me that diagnostic expertise, more than anything else, defines the medical profession. Nowhere is that expertise more important than in EDs. Diagnosis constitutes the bulk of EM practice and permeates every part of it. An ED nurse explained the need for such expertise more bluntly. He said: "Every time a patient comes in with chest pain, all that doctor does is order a cardiac profile. I can do that."

THE WAY US PHYSICIANS ARE EDUCATED AND BECOME BOARD-CERTIFIED PRODUCES A WIDE RANGE OF EXPERTISE

To become a licensed physician, one must graduate from an accredited medical school and pass an exam administered by the National Board of Medical Examiners. To become a board-certified specialist, a doctor must complete several years of related residency training and pass an exam administered by a board of examiners within that specialty. To become a board-certified emergency physician (EM specialist), a doctor must complete three years of EM residency training and pass an exam administered by the American Board of Emergency Medicine (ABEM).

Physicians expend a huge amount of time, money, and effort to acquire a medical education and become board-certified and, therefore, rightly expect that to be enough. The problem is, they're not being well served by a process that hasn't changed much in a hundred years.

After examining the education needed to become a licensed physician, the authors of a 2001 Institute of Medicine (IOM) report to the US Congress concluded: "Despite the changes that have been made, the fundamental approach to clinical education has not changed since 1910."[18] The authors explained that, while curriculum changes are essential, they're not sufficient. Education that focuses on teaching a core of knowledge largely related to basic disease mechanisms and physiologic principles needs to be expanded to teach students how to manage information and use effective tools to support decision-making.

Recent articles and publications continue to call for fundamental changes to medical education.[19, 20, 21, 22, 23] They discuss how changes propelled by the 1910 Flexner Report remain the basis for current education. The Flexner Report transformed medical education in the US and Canada. It called for major changes to how education was funded, the training provided, and the relationship between medical schools and hospitals—changes that firmly established science-based education. These articles call for new changes to address a critical need for better prevention and management of chronic diseases, cost-effective (high-value, low-cost) care, and use of rapidly expanding medical knowledge.

The US board certification process was established in 1933. While the training and tests have changed, to different extents depending on specialty, the process itself has not. And even though the EM certification process was not established until 1980, it's essentially the same as those established earlier. The 2001 IOM report calls for changes to the process to ensure proficiency in evidence-based practice (EBP) and use of decision support tools.[24]

Memorizing enough information to pass a certification exam, much of which can't be recalled three months later, doesn't permit effective use of that info over the next ten years (the usual time period covered by certification). When the certification process was established, physicians had no choice but to process all or most care info from memory only. They do have a choice now, and what needs to be processed has grown exponentially. A 2023 Medscape article summarized the problem: "The amount of medical knowledge is said to double every 73 days, making it much tougher for physicians to identify innovative findings and newer guidelines for helping patients."[25] Current demand for cost-effective care adds a whole new complicated dimension to that.

Continuing medical education (CME), required after a US doctor becomes board-certified, isn't comprehensive or effective enough to ensure appropriate use of needed info over ten years. As noted in the 2001 IOM report, "Traditional methods of continuing education for health professionals, such as formal conferences and dissemination of educational materials, have been shown to have little effect by themselves … Continuing education needs to emphasize a variety of interventions [to ensure correct use of needed info]."[26]

CURRENT DIAGNOSIS-RELATED EDUCATION AND TRAINING IS ESPECIALLY PROBLEMATIC

A 2015 IOM report entitled *Improving Diagnosis in Health Care* calls for specific changes to improve diagnosis. It begins by stating: "The delivery of health care has proceeded for decades with a blind spot: Diagnostic errors—inaccurate or delayed diagnoses—which persist throughout all care settings and continue to harm an unacceptable number of patients."[27]

That report calls for changes related to

- clinical reasoning;
- teamwork;
- communication with patients, their families, and other healthcare professionals;
- appropriate use of diagnostic tests and their results; and
- use of better health IT.

More recent articles and publications call for the same or similar changes to improve diagnosis.[28, 29, 30]

In a 2020 article, the authors begin by stating: "Diagnosis is the cornerstone of providing safe and effective medical care. Still, diagnostic errors are all too common. A key to improving diagnosis in practice is improving diagnosis education, yet formal education about diagnosis is often lacking, idiosyncratic, and not evidence based."[31] It then discusses the need for better education to improve individual performance, teamwork, and system design or implementation.

Chapters 2–4 explain how color-assisted, Bayesian-like analysis can improve diagnosis in all those ways.

THE CURRENT MISDIAGNOSIS RATE IN EDS IS, ITSELF, A BIG PROBLEM

A 2022 study at Johns Hopkins University found a US ED diagnostic error rate of 5.7 percent.[32] It then points out that, given 130 million ED visits per year, that rate translates to 7.4 million diagnostic errors. Those errors harmed 2.5 million patients and caused potentially avoidable death or permanent disability in 350,000 others.

Each of these numbers is greatly exceeded by the number of family members, friends, and others whose lives were disrupted or devastated.

Misdiagnoses or wasteful approaches to diagnosis also contribute to ruinous healthcare spending. As discussed in chapter 5, that spending is bankrupting the US as a whole and millions of its citizens.

Wide-Ranging Diagnostic Expertise Is Also a Major Cause of Physician Burnout

While working in numerous EDs, I found that while some doctors were excellent diagnosticians, many were not, and some were clearly incompetent. Furthermore, even those with great expertise had no way to readily demonstrate it by explaining and justifying a diagnosis when evidenced-based evaluation (and related treatment) failed to prevent a bad outcome—which sometimes happens.

Real or perceived diagnostic incompetence caused the people who interacted with physicians—administrators, nurses, patients, payers, and regulators—to lose respect for their certification. These people therefore tried to control or displace physician practice in ways that demoralized doctors *and made care worse*:

- Administrators let nurses control or displace physician practice.

- Patients demanded and often received care that was costly, potentially harmful, and/or not needed. They were also prompted to expect satisfaction in other ways not related to good care, making doctors more like hospitality workers.

- Payers and regulators tried to control physician practice via meaningful use and shared savings incentives, which greatly compounded the burden of EHR tasks.

- Insurance companies required preapproval for too much care.

Nurse Control or Displacement of Physician Practice Is Especially Problematic

I found such control or displacement of physician practice to be especially demoralizing to doctors and most directly related to their need for a better way to acquire and demonstrate diagnostic expertise.

The following are examples of what I found to be a serious and/or growing problem at nineteen of the twenty-six US EDs where I worked. Again, because diagnosis constitutes the bulk of EM practice and permeates every part of it, the problem was almost always diagnosis related.

SAINT ANNE'S HOSPITAL, FALL RIVER, MASSACHUSETTS

Nurses in this ED were practicing medicine more than I thought possible. Their initial evaluation greatly exceeded usual triage care. They ordered extensive, nonroutine tests. Physicians were told which patients to see and in what order. Furthermore, no doctor was allowed to see any patient until all test results were reported. I often found that the ordered tests were either unnecessary or unhelpful, which resulted in more time being wasted ordering and waiting for results of needed tests. Physician resistance to this practice was futile. In one case, I wasn't allowed to see, even briefly, a child previously seen by another doctor. Before he was discharged, I was instead instructed to view only his test results. Because I read patients better than numbers and was accustomed to doing so, I overlooked a blood urea nitrogen level of 34, indicating dehydration. The patient returned about eighteen hours later, dead and clearly dehydrated. A nurse told me not to worry—the child had a "lousy mother" who ought to be blamed for what happened. I'll never know if the doctor who examined the patient became aware of what happened. I never returned to that ED.

CITY HOSPITAL MARTINSBURG, WEST VIRGINIA

Note: City Hospital is now Berkley Medical Center, part of WVU Health System.

Two weeks after I passed an EM board certification exam and ten minutes into my first shift, a licensed practical nurse with eighteen months of training informed me he had evaluated a patient, decided what that patient needed, and taken admission orders from a psychiatrist. He fully expected me to sign off on that. While I was trying to explain why I wouldn't do so, the psychiatrist entered the ED. He told me to not worry about the patient—he would take care of him. He then discovered the patient didn't need or want to be treated for any psychiatric problem. Despite having a history of chronic schizophrenia, he presented with a specific complaint of back pain. Instead of backtracking and letting me care for that patient, the psychiatrist discharged him and wrote in his note on the ED chart, where my note should have been, "Dr. Sorensen examined him," without letting me do so. I could only hope the patient somehow received needed care for his back pain.

ARNOT OGDEN MEDICAL CENTER, ELMIRA, NEW YORK

A seventy-four-year-old woman had driven her car into a tree after falling asleep. When I began my evaluation of this patient, the nurse involved told me she had already ordered labs, x-rays, and CT scans according to that ED's trauma protocols. A general surgeon at that hospital had reportedly instructed nurses to discharge such patients if their tests, including CT scans, were normal. Because these results were normal, the nurse transferred the patient from the ED to a caretaker's car without telling me. While I was on the phone discussing another patient, the nurse threw a prescription pad in front of me and pounded on it with her finger—her way of telling me to do my job so she could discharge the patient. My evaluation was telling me that, even though the patient's CT scan was normal, her cervical spine was not. She was still complaining of moderately severe neck pain despite several IV doses of analgesics. Also, the pain was worse when she sat up and was associated with point tenderness. Given enough time, I likely would have ordered flexion-extension cervical spine x-rays (I had previously saved a patient's life by doing so as a resident) or at least consulted with that hospital's neurosurgeon. But the patient was already in the car, and I had been conditioned over several years to tolerate such interference, so I didn't do either.

Two days later, the patient returned with persistent neck pain and progressive weakness in her upper extremities. The next day, the admitting neurosurgeon discovered via such x-rays that the patient had an unstable cervical spine (unrestricted movement of C3 over C4) due to torn ligaments not detected by the CT scan. Any additional trauma might well have severed her spinal cord. In response to such working conditions, that ED's medical director had resigned several months previously and was doing only administrative work two days a week. The hospital had been trying to replace him, but without success. For the same reason, two other physicians who had previously been directors didn't want the job. One told me he considered it a bad joke.

ST. JOSEPH'S HOSPITAL, PARKERSBURG, WEST VIRGINIA

The nursing supervisor in this ED was one of the few who insisted that only competent physicians work there *and* made a point of not letting nurses interfere with their practice. Eventually, however, she was fired by an administrator who then "empowered nurses" to better control or displace physician care by doing what nurses were doing in these four, and most other EDs where I worked. All but one physician left. The director reportedly stayed for the sake of his pension.

POCONO MEDICAL CENTER, EAST STROUDSBURG, PENNSYLVANIA

I worked in this ED with the same nurse almost every weekend for nine months. She often expressed respect for and approval of my practice but also seemed quite threatened when I deviated from protocols established by her supervisor—for example, scrubbing a patient's abrasion instead of letting a technician do so. One night, for reasons that seemed quite complicated, she argued with me about and threatened insubordination regarding my every decision. She must have discussed this with her supervisor. Within a week, I was pulled off night shifts, after working those shifts for eight months, and had to work day shifts with another doctor so nurses could control which patients I saw. After three more weekends of escalating interference, I quit.

There are, of course, two sides to these stories. Chapters 2 and 4 describe how both sides might be addressed by giving physicians a better way to acquire and demonstrate diagnostic expertise and using that technology to improve doctor–nurse collaboration.

Physicians Need Better IT to Clearly Establish and Preserve Standard of Care

Variations of the problems I encountered during my practice continue to cause serious physician burnout.

A publication titled "The Reclamation of Emergency Medicine: 'Take EM Back' White Paper," produced by US emergency physicians and updated on July 12, 2021, describes and discusses those problems. It begins by stating: "An emphasis on understaffing and corporate metrics, in combination with a sense of powerlessness to address the ethical transgressions rampant in corporate healthcare, leads to moral injury (formerly known as 'burnout') as emergency physicians are effectively forced to violate their Hippocratic oaths as a condition of employment."[33] In short, corporate profiteering is compromising care and demoralizing doctors. The problems cited include the following:

- private equity (PE) ownership of EM groups and contractual agreements, which result in compromised care

- the proliferation of corporate and PE-funded EM residency programs, which provide insufficient training and produce EM physicians who can be paid less for their service

- notional-only supervision of nonphysician practitioners (NPPs)—requiring one physician to "sign off" on care provided by up to five NPPs per shift, without being allowed to adequately supervise them

- "termination without cause" employment practices permitted by PE-backed management contracts, which prevent physicians from countering ethical transgressions

Those problems seriously threaten physician *and patient* well-being. The American Antitrust Institute recently concluded, "the private equity business model is fundamentally incompatible with a stable, competitive healthcare system that serves patients and promotes the health and wellbeing of the population."[34]

Despite this, emergency physician staffing groups are increasingly being voluntarily sold for exorbitant personal profit or hostilely ousted by PE-backed contract management groups (CMGs). Per *The Reclamation of Emergency Medicine*, by 2021, about 50 percent of US emergency physicians were working for PE-backed CMGs whose profiteering compromises care. [35]

A striking number of doctors are responding by leaving medicine or attempting to do so. The authors of the "Take EM Back" white paper reported finding a Facebook group of physicians seeking alternative employment, a group which touted seventy-nine thousand members.[36] Many others continue working for CMGs only because they see no viable alternative. According to the paper, the 2021 cost of a medical education was $365,000–$440,000.

Physicians need a comprehensive knowledge base containing the best available information, and technology permitting ready and selective access, to clearly establish standard of care and preserve or restore such care which is now being compromised—by legal means if need be. For example, both might be used to

- establish which conditions require physician care and enforce related, appropriate ED staffing,

- improve care of other conditions by NPPs,

- ensure sufficient resident training,

- force CMGs to modify their management of EM practice and related profiteering in other ways, and

- prevent termination without cause, which permits corporate transgressions.

Defining standard of care as that provided by residency-trained, board-certified physicians is not enough for two reasons. Care quality, especially diagnostic, varies greatly among physicians, and that definition isn't nearly specific or detailed enough. It needs to cover established diagnostic criteria and recommended treatment options for each disease. Many thousands of hours have been spent conducting studies to establish both, especially for emergent causes of ED visits. That info isn't being used nearly as well as it could be. For those same reasons, steps taken by regulatory and/or oversight agencies to preserve standard of care—called for by the previously discussed white paper—won't be enough without physician use of such a knowledge base and technology.

All other professionals whose practice is information intensive use IT to preserve practice integrity. Attorneys use LexisNexis and other knowledge bases. The tax version of LexisNexis details what needs to be done to comply with the tax code under every conceivable circumstance. Accountants and other tax professionals must demonstrate proficient use during their education and training. Without use of such IT, they and other professionals wouldn't have a practice. By denying the need for such IT in medicine, many doctors now have a practice they no longer want.

At a recent EM conference, attendees discussed an especially painful reality. Administrators and corporations have been able to largely replace doctor care with nonphysician (NPP) care, partly because patients have not demanded or even requested physician care. Granted, many conditions can be safely managed by NPPs, but those described in the previous section and others discussed at that conference cannot be. Also, wide-ranging expertise or competence is also a problem among NPPs. Given nonphysician (patient) response to the HIPUS® system (described in chapter 7), use of such IT will likely guarantee patient demand for direct care or supervision of NPP care by physicians.

There is certainly a place for the training and testing required for certification, but both need to be modified to facilitate the use of IT over the course of one's practice.

Physicians Need Better IT to Document and Report Care with Greater Ease and Speed

A combination of two factors produced current EHR systems, which are now the number one cause of US physician burnout. During what is often referred to as the EHR gold rush (from about 2009 to 2014), prompted by the US government's decision to reimburse doctors for money spent adopting EHR use,

- physicians demanded EHRs, which required little or no change to how they practiced medicine by trying to process all or most care info, especially diagnostic, from memory only; and

- competing EHR vendors gave doctors what they wanted.

Not long after doctors started using those EHRs, surveys found, many came to hate what they had asked for.

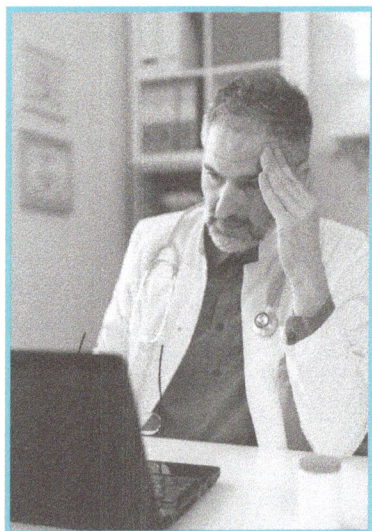

Reasons cited then were the same as those cited in a recent publication:[37]

- information overload

- slow system response times

- excessive data entry

- inability to navigate the system quickly

- note bloat

- fear of missing something

- notes geared toward billing, not patient care

EHR dysfunction also consumes a huge amount of physician time and energy. One study found that *during* office hours, doctors spent about two hours doing EHR-related work for every one hour spent interacting with patients and one to two hours more *after* office hours.[38] Another study found that ED physicians spent 44 percent of their time entering data, compared to 28 percent interacting with patients.[39]

US federal payer and regulator attempts to micromanage physician practice via meaningful use and shared savings incentives (discussed in chapter 5) greatly compounded the burden of performing EHR tasks.

HIPUS® mobile assistance, described in chapters 2 and 6, will let emergency physicians document and report diagnostic care in ways readily understood and likely accepted by payers and regulators with much greater ease and speed. Also, because diagnosis constitutes the bulk of EM practice and permeates every part of it, such assistance can improve and simplify the documenting and reporting of all ED care.

Mobile assistance can be incorporated into any preexisting emergency department information system (EDIS) to let physicians readily collaborate with coworkers, including nurses, technicians, and clerks. I've discussed how that might be done with the founder and president of an EHR vendor that produces systems permitting fully coordinated care by providers in various inpatient and outpatient settings. He recently provided time and cost estimates for incorporating that mobile assistance into his preexisting EDIS of about six months and $500,000. He could then incorporate it into other systems.

The 21st Century Cures Act was enacted by the US Congress in 2016 partly to help make EHRs more useable. It prohibits EHR vendors and others from interfering with the access, exchange, or use of electronic health information and thereby preventing incorporation of new technology into preexisting systems. It also aims to foster an ecosystem of new applications by requiring standardized use of application programming interfaces (APIs).

It can only achieve those objectives, however, if providers—hospitals or physicians— demand the use of new technology. I've found hospitals have little incentive to do so. As explained in this chapter, physicians have ample reasons to demand new technology but (as discussed in chapter 7) fear necessary change too much to do so.

CHAPTER 2

Burnout—The Solution

THIS CHAPTER DESCRIBES how use of better IT can address physician burnout and improve patient care by letting doctors more easily acquire and demonstrate diagnostic expertise, document and report care with greater ease and speed, and clearly establish and enforce standard of care. It also describes how the use of such IT greatly improved and benefited my own practice.

Letting Physicians More Easily Acquire and Demonstrate Diagnostic Expertise

To diagnose competently and cost-effectively, a physician needs to know

- which diseases to consider,

- which findings (signs, symptoms, and test results) to look for, and

- the significance of the presence (specificity) and/or absence (sensitivity) of findings in ruling in or out each disease.

Numerous textbooks and journal articles call for thorough, systematic use of findings, especially history and physical. Two notable examples are:

"An organized approach to a patient with chest pain is essential, to ensure that all causes are evaluated appropriately. The history and physical examination are key to diagnosis. Information pertinent to the differential diagnosis is obtained through the history, physical examination, and [electrocardiogram] ECG in 80 to 90 percent of patients." —James E. Brown, MD, author, "Chest Pain" chapter, *Rosen's Emergency Medicine: Concepts and Clinical Practice*, 9th Edition.

"The necessity of making a thorough physical examination in every acute abdominal case should not need much emphasis. Radiologic or ultrasonic examinations, CT scans, and the vast array of laboratory tests available to all of us today will not compensate for a poor or incomplete history and physical examination." —William Silen, MD, author, *Cope's Early Diagnosis of the Acute Abdomen* (revised), 21st Edition.

Bayesian statistical analysis permits consideration of all needed info—not only all diseases that might cause a condition and a complete set of history and physical findings needed to rule each in or out, but also the prevalence of each disease in a given population (or incidence in ED patients) and the significance of the presence (specificity) and/or absence (sensitivity) of every finding (history, physical, test result) in ruling in or out each disease. During such analysis, disease likelihood is calculated using disease prevalence or incidence and finding sensitivity and/or specificity for each disease. Both are crucial determinants of disease likelihood. A rare disease is much less likely than a very common disease, even if the findings found to be present or absent are equally specific or sensitive for both diseases.

Bayesian analysis uses the following formula to calculate disease likelihood using disease prevalence or incidence and finding specificity and/or sensitivity.

$$p(\theta|D) = \frac{p(D|\theta)p(\theta)}{p(D)} \propto p(D|\theta)p(\theta)$$

Don't be scared off by this formula. You don't need to understand it—whether you're a doctor or not. For now, you only need to know the following:

- Disease incidence is a measure of how frequently a disease occurs in a specified population over a period of time. For example, in a given year, how many people who go to a particular ED are having a heart attack?

- Finding specificity is a measure of how often a disease is present, given the presence of a finding. For example, what percentage of ED patients who present with chest pain are having a heart attack?

- Finding sensitivity is a measure of how often a finding is present, given the presence of a disease. For example, what percentage of ED patients who are having a heart attack present with chest pain?

In 1972, F.T. de Dombal and his colleagues demonstrated successful use of the formula to evaluate acute abdominal pain. Average diagnostic accuracy was 91.5 percent with use, compared to 72.2 percent for surgeons without. Accuracy among ED physicians without was 40–45 percent.[40, 41]

Francis Timothy de Dombal, born August 16, 1937, in Sheffield, England, was a man of enormous energy and intellect. He was a surgeon, accomplished jazz pianist, race car driver, and astronomer. At an early age, he turned his attention to computerized data collection and retrieval to improve diagnostic accuracy. While serving as chair of the World Congress of Gastroenterology Research Committee, he directed multinational studies in both developed and newly emerging nations. His groundbreaking use of Bayesian statistical analysis prompted widespread use of Bayesian systems by demonstrating the importance of using disease prevalence or incidence and related finding specificity/sensitivity, thoroughly and systematically, when ruling in or out possible diagnoses.

Use of the aforementioned formula, however, is quite complicated and foreign to the way physicians think about diagnosis. Doctors, therefore, are largely locked out of the diagnostic process when using a Bayesian system. The system is a black box. The physician can only input findings and receive the system's concluded diagnosis without being able to control how those findings are processed or explain and justify that diagnosis to others.

The HIPUS® System

By using *colors* to convey the specificity and/or sensitivity of findings for each disease, the HIPUS® system overcomes the "black box" problem with Bayesian systems and allows physicians to more easily acquire and demonstrate diagnostic expertise by letting them

- more easily *learn and recall* what they need to know,

- *fully* process that info at the bedside, and

- readily *explain and justify* diagnostic and related decisions to others.

The following sections describe how this might be done.

USE FOR STUDY

Dr. James Brown, who authored the "Chest Pain" chapter in *Rosen's Emergency Medicine: Concepts and Clinical Practice* (9th edition), emphasized the need for systematic use of history, physical, and other findings when evaluating chest pain. Emergent causes (those that require or may require hospitalization) include:

- acute myocardial infarction (AMI; also known as heart attack),

- unstable (new or worsening) angina (UA),

- aortic dissection (tearing of the aortic wall in the chest),

- spontaneous pneumothorax (partial lung collapse),

- pulmonary embolism (movement of part of a blood clot from a leg or other vein to the artery supplying blood to one or both lungs),

- pneumonia (infection involving one or both lungs),

- acute pericarditis (painful inflammation of the sac surrounding the heart), and

- esophageal rupture (permitting movement of esophageal/stomach content into the chest cavity).

These disorders cause overlapping symptoms, signs, and test results. Each, however, causes a characteristic or distinguishing *combination* of findings. Each can be ruled in or out using the specificity and/or sensitivity of those findings.

The next images show how the HIPUS® system uses colors to present the diagnostic profile (characteristic findings) for acute pericarditis.

Color coding

Purple if present **help rule out**

Green if present **are diagnostic**

Orange and yellow findings are listed in decreasing order of sensitivity. Orange always or almost always occur--yellow, less often. Therefore:

Orange if *absent* **help rule out** if present **help rule in**

Yellow if absent don't help much if present **add support to orange**

Secondary colors add to / modify the meanings of primary colors. Their meaning can be accessed by tapping on the symbols.

An X says more about *absence* A ● or O more about *presence*

Pericarditis

Negative CMR or CCT

Criteria (two or more)
X **Chest pain**
   Sharp or stabbing/pleuritic
   Relieved by sitting and
      leaning forward
   Aggravated by lying supine
X **Pericardial friction rub**
X **ECG: widespread ST elevation and PR depression**
X **Pericardial effusion per TTE or CXR**

Additional supportive criteria
   CCT: enhanced pericardium
   CMR: pericardial edema, late
      gadolinium enhancement

Elevated inflammation marker:
   WBC, ESR / CRP

The color-coding scheme used to convey the significance of the presence or absence (specificity or sensitivity) of the findings for acute pericarditis is presented on the first screen. As shown, physicians need to remember the meanings of only four primary (main) colors. The meanings of secondary colors can be quickly accessed by tapping on the symbols. For an explanation of the secondary colors, see page 2.

As shown in the following images …

< Pericarditis	< Statements
Negative CMR or CCT	**Negative CMR** or CCT

Criteria (two or more)
X Chest pain
   Sharp or stabbing/pleuritic
   Relieved by sitting and
     leaning forward
   Aggravated by lying supine
X Pericardial friction rub
**X ECG: widespread ST eleva-
   tion and PR depression**
**X Pericardial effusion per
   TTE or CXR**
	Should it be necessary to rule out pericarditis, cardiac magnetic resonance (CMR) can do so more reliably than cardiac computed tomography (CCT) due to its superior ability to distinguish normal from inflamed pericardial tissue—sensitivity is 94-100%. [1,2]

Additional supportive criteria
   CCT: enhanced pericardium
   CMR: pericardial edema, late
     gadolinium enhancement
	Criteria (two or more)...
	
	Pericarditis is defined as inflammation of the pericardium with or without effusion. The diagnosis can be established using any two criteria: characteristic chest pain, pericardial friction rub, typical ECG pattern, and new or worsening pericardial effusion. [1]

Elevated inflammation marker: WBC, ESR / CRP	**X Chest pain: Sharp or stabbing and/or pleuritic; relieved by sitting and leaning forward; ag-**

… each finding (first screen) is linked to one or more statements (second screen), which describe and/or discuss its specificity/sensitivity. Each statement is linked to one or more supporting sources by the red numbers shown. Statements reinforce and add to the meanings of the colors. The findings can be viewed or reviewed, almost at a glance, and then used to quickly study or review related statements. Over time, most findings and statements can be recalled without review.

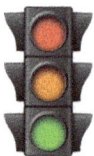

The HIPUS® system's use of colors was granted patent protection because, like traffic signals, it gives physicians lifesaving info without their having to even think about the meanings of the colors, which, in turn, lets them fully process that info whenever needed.

Dr. Carol Rivers, who edited and published preparatory textbooks for EM board exams, strongly endorsed use of this color-coded interface in a letter addressed to my patent attorney.

She stated, in part: "Color coding data allows the user to learn more (and remember more) so that, with repeated use, he not only increases his knowledge base but also becomes more sophisticated (academically and clinically) in the decision-making process. In other words, by using the program, the physician becomes more astute in his clinical practice."

In an article titled "The influence of colour on memory performance: a review," Mariam Dzulkifli and her colleague reviewed several studies that found use of colors increases short- and long-term recall of info by increasing human attention and emotional arousal in response to its presentation.[42]

The person who helped design HIPUS® bedside assistance is color-blind and helped create schemes to accommodate color blindness.

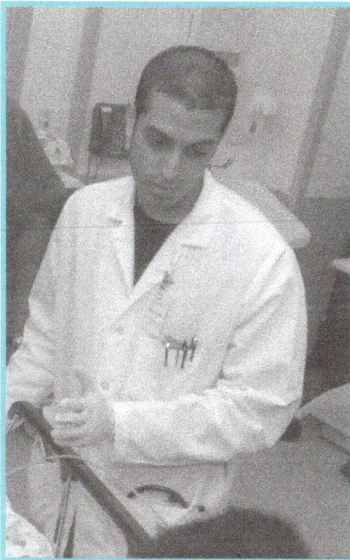

USE AT THE BEDSIDE

After using profile findings and related statements for study or review, if a doctor then, at the bedside,

- identifies the patient's chief complaint,

- asks up to eight related questions covering location, quality, quantity, onset, course, precipitating event, alleviating or aggravating factors, and/or associated symptoms,

- performs a related physical exam, and

- views routine lab, ECG, and/or X-ray results, he can usually identify the correct diagnosis or select possibilities from a list.

He can then use corresponding checklist findings, along with profile findings and statements, to quickly

- rule each diagnosis in or out,

- document doing so, and/or

- explain and justify doing so to others.

After asking up to eight open-ended questions and listening to the answers carefully, using a mobile device and checklist findings to ask follow-up questions will likely inspire not less but more patient confidence.

The HIPUS® system is designed to improve study and bedside use of diagnostic info in two other ways (discussed further in chapter 3).

It treats disease *variations* as separate diagnostic entities to help a doctor avoid overlooking a diagnosis and/or focus on crucial related information. For example, the variations of AMI (heart attack) are presented separately as AMI: typical, AMI: painless, and AMI: young patient. The system lets a doctor study those variations and then, at the bedside, safely select the one that needs to be considered. Ruling in or out a variation (e.g., AMI: young patient) rules in or out the disease (i.e., AMI).

It also facilitates what I found to be the most sure-footed approach to diagnosis, especially in EDs. That approach consists of

- identifying the patient's chief complaint—the *main* reason for seeking care (e.g., shortness of breath),

- determining the *primary and direct* cause of that complaint (e.g., congestive heart failure),

- ruling in or out other diseases known to occur along with that direct cause (e.g., AMI), and

- repeating the previous steps for any finding (symptom, sign, test result) discovered and not yet explained (e.g., knee pain).

Treatment info will be presented for study using *menu items*, statements and sources, and at the bedside in various ways—for example, as a list of recommended drugs needed to provide and report care.

The use of free or unrestricted dictation to cover the unique or unusual aspects of any case will permit use of checklist findings and other care data without restricting or oversimplifying care. Data generated via free dictation will be used to improve the knowledge base over time.

> *In short, combined use of profile findings, checklist findings, and free dictation is essential for solving not only physician burnout but also uneven care quality and out-of-control costs (discussed in chapters 5 and 6). The system will need to be tested and refined several times to optimize combined use of those findings and free dictation, and physician time and effort will be needed to master its use. But the benefits of doing both will far outweigh the costs.*

Most HIPUS® system attributes are those called for by the 2015 IOM report.

The IOM 2015 report, *Improving Diagnosis in Health Care* (discussed in chapter 1), includes recommendations for improving related IT and discusses the following key attributes of safe, effective IT:

- easy retrieval of accurate, timely, and reliable data

- simple and intuitive data displays

- easy navigation

- evidence at the point of care to aid decision-making

- enhancements to workflow—automating mundane tasks and minimizing cognitive workload[43]

Websites at hipus.study and hipus.care provide access to a demo prototype and slideshows that describe how those attributes make HIPUS® system use easy, safe, and effective. Because the demo and shows were created as a basis for building applications, they might present more detail than you want to study. When viewing the demo at hipus.study, I recommend moving through all the screens quickly to see how the system is used for study and then going back to study screen content if you want to do so. Each slideshow (with voice-over) at hipus.care can be easily viewed in about three to five minutes. Viewing the first two will give you a good idea of how bedside assistance works.

The following images show how the system permits easy navigation.

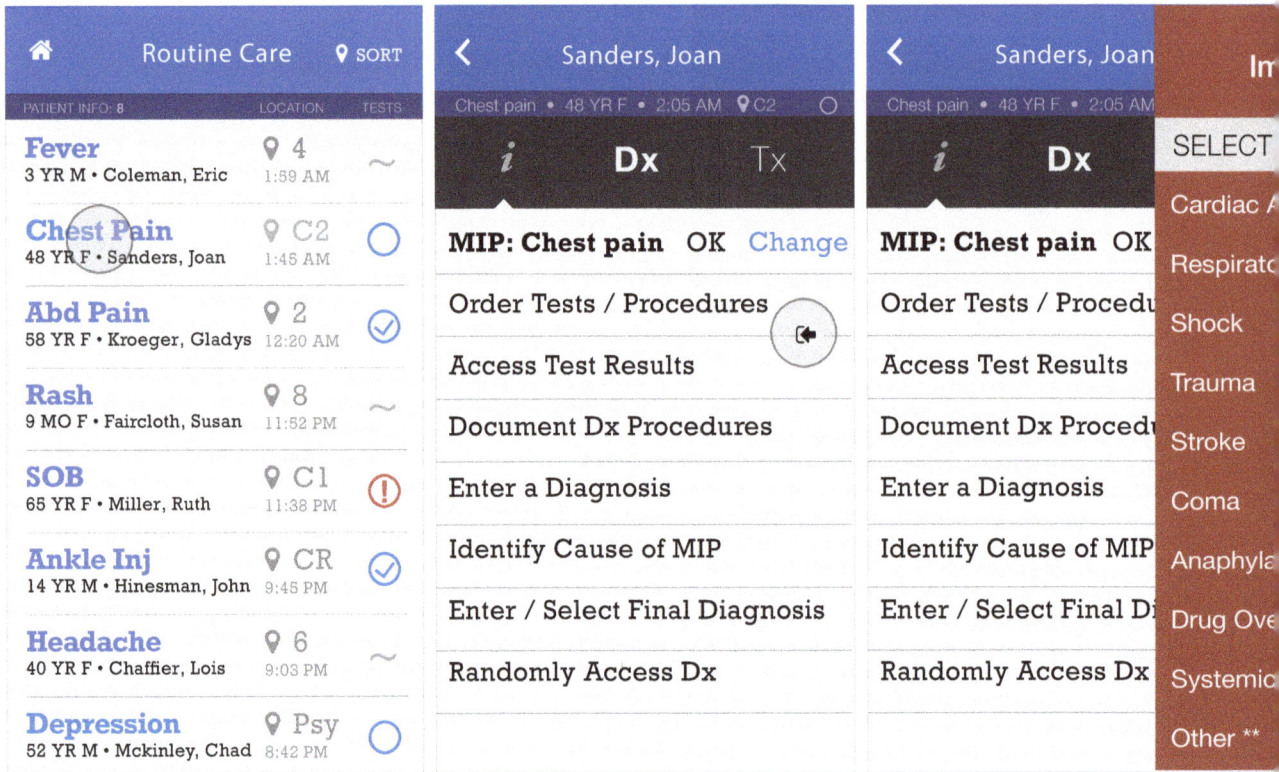

After accessing the bedside assistance app, the ED physician uses the Routine Care menu (first screen) to view a list of his current patients. When the physician selects Joan Sanders with a chief complaint of chest pain (entered by the triage nurse), the system lets him use the drop-down menu at the top of the next screen to access any of three menus: patient info (*i*), diagnosis (Dx), or treatment (Tx).

Selecting the diagnosis menu lets the physician *first* accept or change that chief complaint (main/initial presentation) and download all related care data (not shown). After he does that, the system presents the menu shown, which he can use to perform any listed task.

At any time, while using that or any menu provided by the system, touching anywhere on the screen and swiping left (◀) brings up a menu (next screen) that lets the physician manage a cardiac arrest or any condition requiring immediate care and document doing so.

Use of the Routine Care (patient), drop-down, and Immediate Care menus lets the physician quickly move from one point in the system to another and return to any, while caring for several patients simultaneously.

Letting Physicians Document and Report Care with Greater Ease and Speed

The following describes how the HIPUS® system might be used to document and report evaluation of chest pain in Joan Sanders given two different scenarios.

In the first scenario, after identifying the patient's chief complaint, asking the aforementioned eight questions, performing a related physical exam, and viewing the patient's ECG and chest x-ray (ordered by the nurse per an established protocol), the physician is reasonably certain that acute pericarditis is the cause of Joan's chest pain and sees no need to consider other possibilities.

Therefore, he selects "Enter a Diagnosis" on the Dx menu. Using a series of steps, he then indicates the presence or absence of checklist findings for that disease and then indicates that acute pericarditis is his concluded diagnosis.

The system then lets him document, report, and explain that concluded diagnosis when it generates a record of that ED care episode. It does so using the doctor's dictated summary of the episode covering the most important, unique, and/or unusual aspects of the case; color-coded profile findings found to be present or absent (using corresponding checklist findings); and results of ordered tests used to determine the presence or absence of certain profile findings.

The following images show how a different physician, while caring for the same patient in the same ED, three months later, might view that record.

Routine Care • SORT

PATIENT INFO: 8	LOCATION	TESTS

Fing laceration
18 YR M • Brady, Jack — 4 — 6:03 PM — ~

Headache
23 YR F • Sanchez, Millie — 6 — 5:47 PM — ~

Chest Pain
48 YR F • Sanders, Joan — C1 — 5:14 PM — ○

Dysuria
29 YR F • Freeman, Rose — 8 — 4:52 PM — ✓

Earache
6 YR M • Ling, Chen — Ped — 4:38 PM — ~

Epigastric pain
14 YR M • Rhoads, John — 3 — 3:45 PM — ✓

< Sanders, Joan

Chest pain • 48 YR F • 2:05 AM • C2 ○

i   Dx   Tx

Admission and Billing

Triage

Medical History

  Established Diagnoses

ED Care

  05/14/2022 **H**IPUS

  12/06/2016

  OTHER **

Hospitalizations

< Sanders, Joan

ED Care: 05/14/2022

Summary

Diagnosis ....

  Findings

  ECG

  Lab, X-ray

Treatment **

Response **

Disposition **

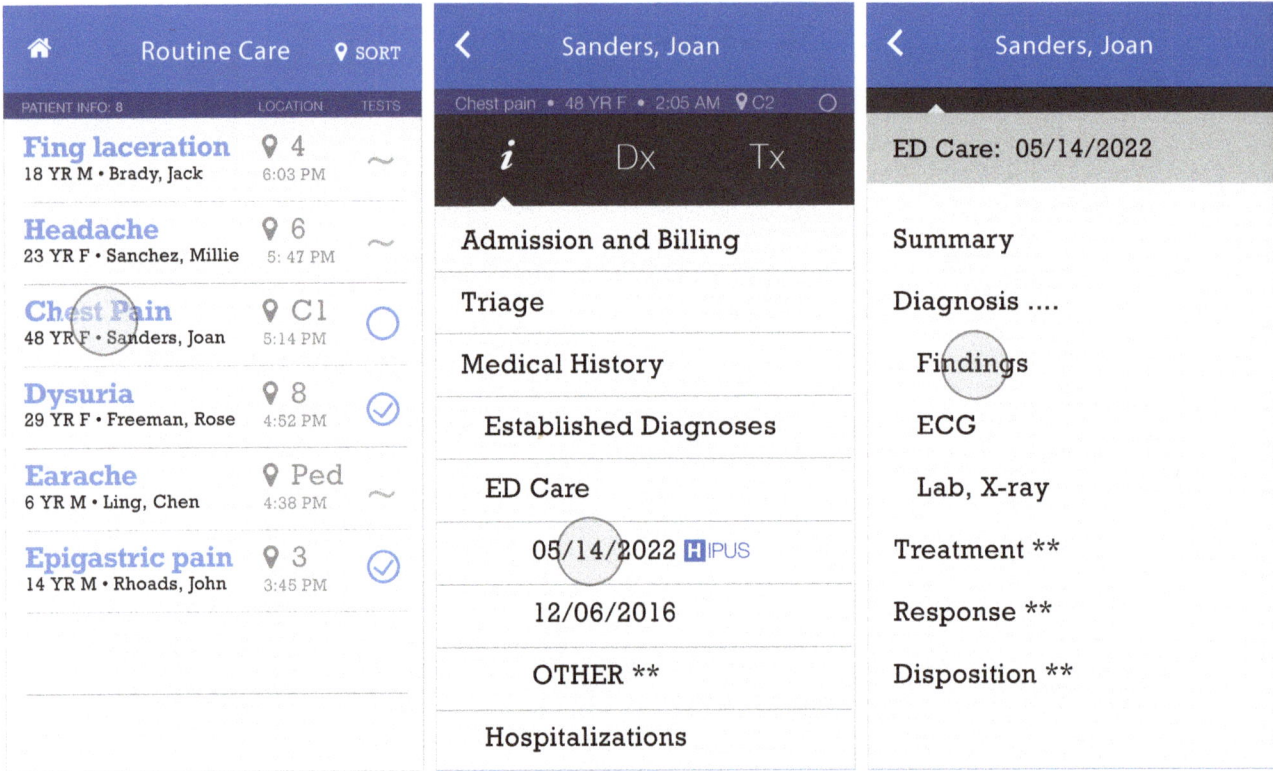

Joan Sanders has returned due to chest pain recurrence. The physician initiates or resumes care of Mrs. Sanders using the Routine Care menu.

After doing so, she uses the patient info (*i*) menu to access the record of previous care by selecting that ED care episode from the patient's entire medical record. The logo indicates that this ED record, unlike previous ones, was produced using the HIPUS® system.

Using the last screen, after reading the care summary dictated by the previous doctor (not shown), the physician accesses diagnosis-related info by first tapping on "Diagnosis" and then on "Findings."

As the following images show …

Screen 1:

‹ Sanders, Joan

Diagnosis: Acute pericarditis

Findings present...   View ECG

Criteria: two or more ...
 Chest pain
  Sharp or stabbing/pleuritic
  Relieved by sitting and
   leaning forward
  Aggravated by lying supine
 **ECG: widespread ST eleva-
 tion and PR depression**
Elevated inflammation marker:
WBC

Findings absent...

X Pericardial friction rub
X Pericardial effusion

Findings not found to be
present or absent **

Screen 2:

‹ Sanders, Joan

Diagnosis: Acute pericarditis

View Lab, X-ray

Screen 3:

‹ Sanders, Joan

Diagnosis: Acute pericarditis

Lab results

WBC	**19.8 H**	NEUT	63.9 %
RBC	4.39	LYMPH	25.4 %
HGB	14.2	MONO	9.0 %
HCT	41.7	EOS	1.3O
PLT	263 K	BASO	0.4 %

OTHER **

**To view x-ray on large screen
tap** here

… the physician sees that the diagnosis was concluded using the needed presence of only two criteria (green sub-findings), despite the absence of others, which were not needed. The physician can also view findings not found to be present or absent—findings, in this case, not needed to rule in or out acute pericarditis. After viewing the findings used to conclude that diagnosis, the physician views the ECG, lab test result, and x-ray used to determine the presence or absence of certain findings by tapping on the links in the right upper corner of the first two screens, or returning to, and using the previously described 05/14/2022 ED care episode menu.

The red font on the last screen highlights the *lab result* used to determine the presence of the *finding* "Elevated inflammation marker: WBC" shown on the first screen. The presence of that finding supports, but is not needed to establish, the diagnosis. It's actually a yellow finding in the diagnostic profile for acute pericarditis but is presented here using black font because orange and yellow indicate sensitivity or frequency of occurrence. When orange and yellow findings are *present*, their frequency of occurrence is irrelevant.

33

The physician can access other info about that care episode (treatment, patient response, etc.) using the ED care episode menu. How non-diagnostic care is documented and reported is described at hipus.care and elsewhere via other slideshows.

In this second scenario, Mrs. Sanders's pain is characteristic of acute pericarditis, but her ECG is not. The physician also finds no pericardial friction rub per physical exam and no effusion per imaging study. He is therefore less certain of that diagnosis. Also, the patient has several heart attack risk factors—smoking, high blood pressure, and high cholesterol. Generally, the presence or absence of risk factors isn't nearly as helpful in ruling in or out a diagnosis as that of findings *caused* by that disease, but the presence of several risk factors warrants consideration of it. Using the Diagnosis menu, the physician therefore selects "Identify cause of M/I Presentation" and then works through the checklist findings for not only acute pericarditis but also heart attack with typical symptoms and unstable angina. As shown on the following pages, he then uses the HIPUS® system to rule each in or out,

document doing so, and explain and justify doing so to others.

The physician uses the Bayesian menu shown here to consider the implications of his checklist-related entries. Slideshows at hipus.care explain all the text and symbols and detail use of each.

For now, disease name abbreviations are presented in the top row. The bars represent profile findings linked to corresponding checklist findings. Findings above the line were found to be present—those below, absent. Black bars represent orange or yellow findings found to be present (again, when present, their sensitivity or frequency of occurrence is irrelevant). The bars at the bottom represent findings whose presence or absence has not yet been determined.

As shown in the following images, the physician chooses to first consider AMI: typical.

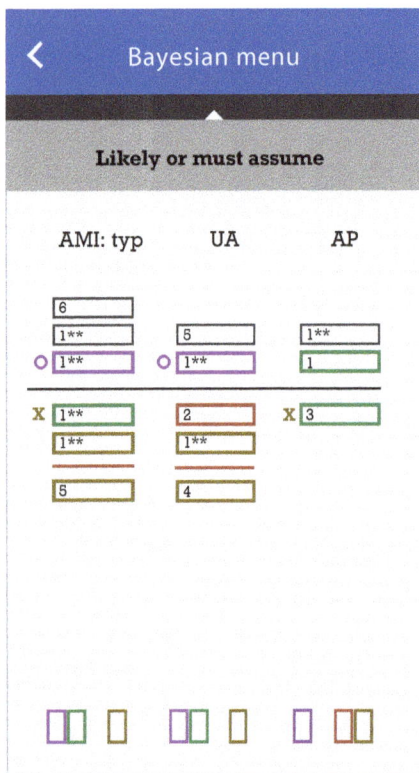

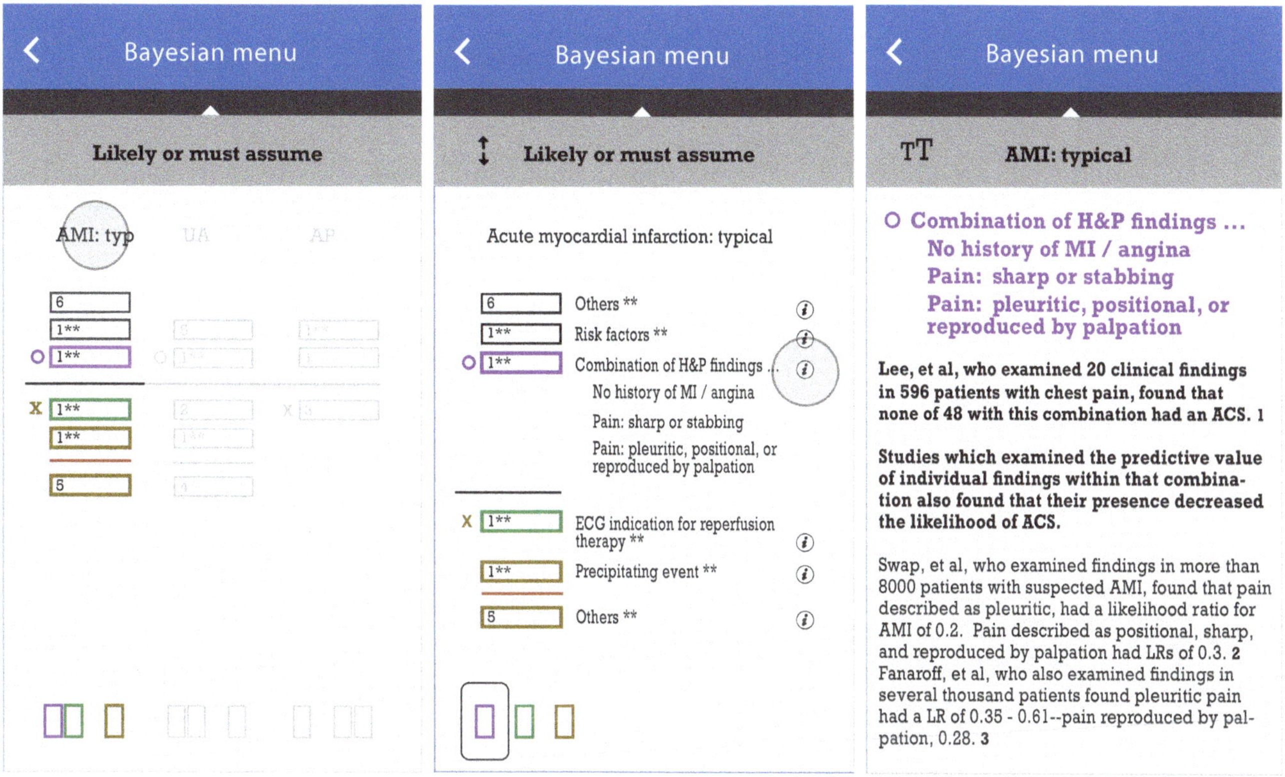

On the first screen, the numbers in each bar indicate the number of findings represented. The double asterisk (**) tells the physician that finding is a *composite* finding with more than one *sub-finding*. The purple bar and *circle* represent a composite finding whose presence makes AMI unlikely but doesn't rule it out (purple *dot* definitely rules out). The physician chooses to learn more about that finding by tapping on "AMI: typ," which lets him view the *names* of the findings found to be present or absent. Expanding that purple composite finding shows the sub-findings. The physician then reviews HIPUS® knowledge base statements linked to that finding by tapping on the info icon.

On the last screen, those statements describe four studies that support use of that finding to help rule out an acute coronary syndrome—AMI *and* UA. The purple bar at the bottom of the second screen indicates that the presence of other purple findings can be used to more or less rule out AMI: typ. After using certain purple findings to definitely rule out AMI and UA, the physician turns his attention to acute pericarditis. As shown next …

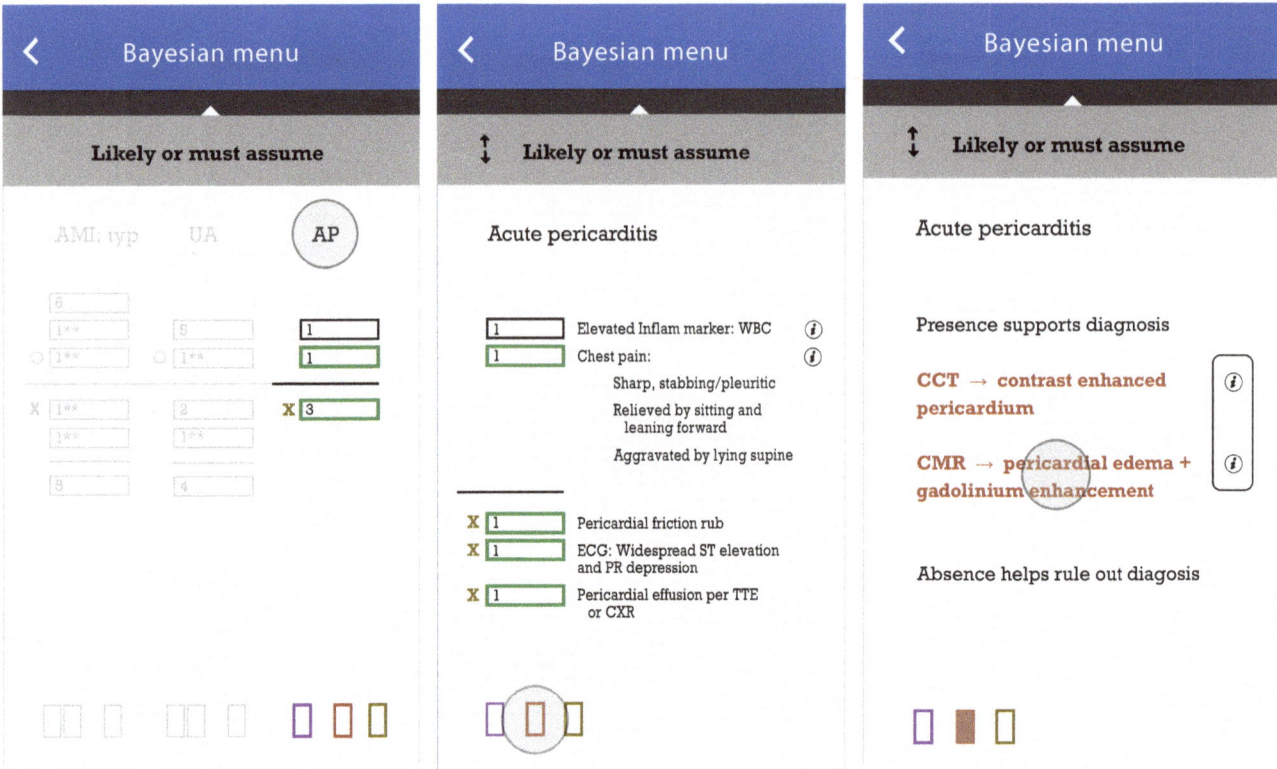

Bayesian menu

Likely or must assume

AMI. typ   UA   AP

8
1**   5
1**   1**

X 1**   2   X 3
1**   1**
9   4

Bayesian menu

Likely or must assume

Acute pericarditis

1   Elevated Inflam marker: WBC   *(i)*
1   Chest pain: *(i)*
      Sharp, stabbing/pleuritic
      Relieved by sitting and
      leaning forward
      Aggravated by lying supine

X 1   Pericardial friction rub
X 1   ECG: Widespread ST elevation
      and PR depression
X 1   Pericardial effusion per TTE
      or CXR

Bayesian menu

Likely or must assume

Acute pericarditis

Presence supports diagnosis

**CCT → contrast enhanced
pericardium**   *(i)*

**CMR → pericardial edema +
gadolinium enhancement**   *(i)*

Absence helps rule out diagosis

… tapping on "AP" (first screen) lets him view the names of present and absent findings (next screen).

The orange bar at the bottom indicates that the not-yet-determined presence or absence of one or more findings can help rule in *or out* acute pericarditis. Tapping on that bar reveals the names of those findings (last screen).

Black text reinforces the meaning of orange. The physician then uses the info icons to access statements about the tests used to determine the presence or absence of each finding. He therefore decides to order a cardiac magnetic resonance scan by tapping on the finding. Performing that test confirms the presence of the finding. While waiting for the results, he can easily initiate or resume care of one or more other patients. After viewing the results …

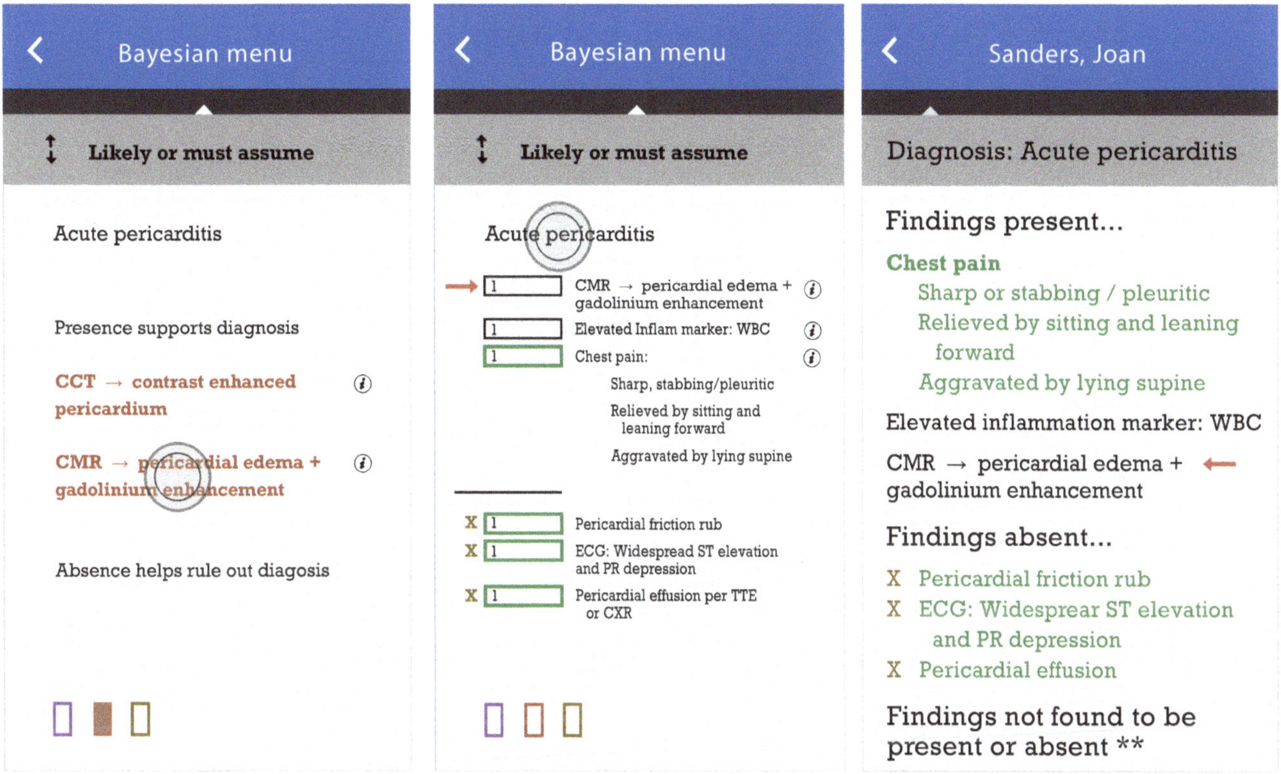

Screen 1:

< Bayesian menu

↕ **Likely or must assume**

Acute pericarditis

Presence supports diagnosis

CCT → contrast enhanced pericardium (i)

CMR → pericardial edema + gadolinium enhancement (i)

Absence helps rule out diagosis

▢ ▢ ▢

Screen 2:

< Bayesian menu

↕ **Likely or must assume**

Acute pericarditis

→ [1] CMR → pericardial edema + (i)
gadolinium enhancement

[1] Elevated Inflam marker: WBC (i)

[1] Chest pain: (i)

Sharp, stabbing/pleuritic

Relieved by sitting and
leaning forward

Aggravated by lying supine

X [1] Pericardial friction rub

X [1] ECG: Widespread ST elevation
and PR depression

X [1] Pericardial effusion per TTE
or CXR

▢ ▢ ▢

Screen 3:

< Sanders, Joan

Diagnosis: Acute pericarditis

Findings present...

Chest pain
Sharp or stabbing / pleuritic
Relieved by sitting and leaning
forward
Aggravated by lying supine

Elevated inflammation marker: WBC

CMR → pericardial edema + ←
gadolinium enhancement

Findings absent...

X Pericardial friction rub

X ECG: Widesprear ST elevation
and PR depression

X Pericardial effusion

**Findings not found to be
present or absent ***

… the physician can quickly return to that screen and indicate the presence of that finding by tapping *and holding* on its name.

When the physician returns to the next screen, he sees that the system has added that name to others presented previously (→). Having ruled out AMI and UA, the physician now considers the presence of acute pericarditis likely enough to warrant related treatment and indicates that by tapping and holding on its name.

As shown on the last screen, the system then presents the diagnosis and the findings used to conclude it within the record of that ED care episode.

The physician could also view the findings used to rule out AMI: typical and UA (not shown).

Letting Physicians Clearly Establish and Enforce Standard of Care

The same IT that lets physicians more easily acquire and demonstrate diagnostic expertise can also be used to establish and enforce standard of care.

Data organized around color-coded diagnostic data will let physicians more easily construct, maintain, and use the required knowledge base. By collaborating with the ABEM, which administers certification exams, an EM professional organization can likely construct a comprehensive knowledge base within five years. A knowledge base covering only the following ED presentations could be constructed in less than two years and used to produce a marketable product that benefits those physicians financially:

- AMI presentations (chest pain, dyspnea/shortness of breath, and, to a limited degree, uncommon or rare presentations)

- abdominal pain

- headache

Over time, *updating* knowledge base content will constitute the vast majority of what needs to be done. Large language model (LLM) technology, described in chapter 3, will let physicians perform this task with much greater ease and speed.

After working with nonphysicians over several years, I and several collaborators are now fully prepared to implement all needed technology.

Use of that knowledge base and technology can be expanded over time without disrupting how physicians currently earn CME credits, prepare for board exams, and interact with patients. This won't solve the problems discussed in chapter 1 overnight, but knowing there is a solution and working toward it can, itself, address burnout.

Creation and Use of Color-Coded Diagnostic Profiles for Study Greatly Improved and Benefited My Own Practice

After residency training, as preparation for my work on this project and continuous work in EDs, I spent two years studying the diagnosis of 150 causes of abdominal pain, thirty causes of chest pain, and twenty causes of headache and creating color-coded diagnostic profiles conveying finding specificity and/or sensitivity for each disease variation. Doing so was many times more helpful than study by any other means. It worked the way Dr. Carol Rivers said it would and was 100 percent relevant to the lion's share of my practice.

Focusing on diagnosis greatly improved and simplified my practice. I found that, after concluding a diagnosis, treatment was obvious, established by protocol, determined in part by the admitting or consulting physician, and/or needed info could be readily accessed via sources such as *The Sanford Guide to Antimicrobial Therapy*. A mobile device could be used to quickly recall any needed treatment info.

Studying history and physical findings was especially helpful. By using those findings alone, I was able to quickly diagnose and successfully treat or manage several life-threatening disorders. As in the case of meningococcal meningitis described in the introduction, in the following cases I needed to use only a few findings to do so. I was therefore troubled to discover that the way US physicians are educated and become board-certified failed to prepare several colleagues to do the same.

- A middle-aged male patient came to the ED after sustaining a stab wound next to the lower left side of his sternum. To me, the diagnosis was obvious—cardiac tamponade (failure of the heart to expand enough to pump needed blood) caused by that stabbing, which penetrated the sac around his heart and allowed blood to fill it. I quickly realized this because of the patient's very low systolic blood pressure (50 mm/Hg), distended neck veins (due to venous blood backing up into his neck), and normal breath sounds bilaterally, which told me his lungs hadn't been damaged (the alternative explanation). Performing immediate pericardiocentesis (inserting a needle into the sac and aspirating the blood from around his heart) caused the man's blood pressure to jump to 150 mm/Hg and saved his life. A colleague, who was also present when the patient arrived, clearly didn't suspect that diagnosis and instead suggested ordering a chest x-ray for no explained reason.

- A woman in her mid-thirties came to the ED a few days after giving birth to her infant daughter with a chief complaint of severe pain in the area around her vaginal orifice. My examination revealed a fairly large (12–15 cm), indurated (stiff and swollen), and very tender area involving the skin and underlying tissue in that area. She also had a low-grade fever. To me, that combination of findings clearly indicated the presence of a serious postpartum infection. During a phone conversation, I learned that her obstetrician believed the patient's pain was due to an allergic reaction. I presented the case for infection given the presence of the previously described findings and absence of those usually caused by an allergic reaction (itching, a raised red rash that is not or only mildly tender, and no fever). By doing so, I persuaded that doctor to admit the patient and assumed she would then examine the area herself and treat it as a serious infection. Instead, either she or her resident examined the patient and, after doing so, treated the area as an allergic reaction with only steroids, which accelerated spread of the infection. Sixteen hours later the patient died of necrotizing fasciitis, a rapidly advancing skin and soft tissue infection that causes widespread necrosis (death) of muscle, fascia, and subcutaneous tissue.

- A young woman presented with left-sided pelvic pain after missing two periods. During the previous week, *three* pelvic ultrasounds failed to show an ectopic (tubal) pregnancy. The presence of several history and physical findings however, including pelvic pain, her report of irregular, scant, and dark vaginal bleeding, and a tender left-sided pelvic mass, along with a positive pregnancy test, indicated high likelihood of ectopic pregnancy. The patient reluctantly agreed to be hospitalized. The next day, laparoscopy (viewing the pelvic cavity by inserting a scope through the lower abdominal wall) confirmed the diagnosis. In this case, the gynecologist who ordered those ultrasounds clearly suspected an ectopic pregnancy and, fortunately, performed that laparoscopy rather than using those ultrasounds to rule it out. My experience tells me more than a few other physicians might have relied on those ultrasounds.

The following describes a lifesaving diagnosis I missed due to overreliance on the absence of cough and fever and presence of a normal chest x-ray. An elderly male presented with a chief complaint of flu-like symptoms and a blood pressure of 80 mm/Hg. I assumed that the latter was due to dehydration and therefore initiated treatment by administering only normal saline intravenously. Doing so failed to raise his blood pressure and instead produced signs of shock, including altered mental status (confusion), rapid heart rate, weak pulse, and low urine output. I therefore assumed the cause was likely infection rather than hypovolemia (inadequate blood volume). Because I found no source for such an infection, I administered a broad-spectrum antibiotic, which also failed to reverse his condition and, over the next several hours, led to his death. That experience prompted me to review the causes, presentation, and treatment of septic shock. I thereby learned that one fatal cause is penicillin-resistant pneumococcal pneumonia, which quickly causes shock without producing clinical evidence of pneumonia and must be treated with a more effective antibiotic regimen than those normally used for pneumonia. The set of useful findings in such cases are advanced age, perhaps male gender, malaise or flu-like symptoms, low blood pressure with or without shock, and non-response to fluid therapy. Later, knowing that helped me save other patients who presented in similar ways.

My diagnostic skills benefited my practice in several ways. Usually, when I quit working in a problematic ED (described in chapter 1), I was offered more money to work elsewhere. My hourly pay rate more than tripled over ten years. One placement agent I worked with while doing locum tenens work said to me, "Most of the doctors we send there are not invited back, but you can stay there forever." I often received such feedback. In several EDs, colleagues invited me into their homes, fed me, and wooed me in other ways. The director of a level II trauma center pretty much put together my application to sit for a board certification exam because he wanted me to stay. My aptitude for EM practice surely contributed to my success, but my diagnostic prowess was the critical factor.

Creation and use of a diagnostic profile also prevented a malpractice lawsuit that my insurer at first considered a certainty. The case involved a diagnosis I may or may not have missed. While I was working at a hospital in West Virginia, the ED director informed me that a patient I had cared for went to another hospital two days later with a ruptured appendix and a senior claims representative with our malpractice insurer planned to meet with me because she fully expected related litigation. During that meeting, I showed her the color-coded diagnostic profile I created for appendicitis and the sources used to create it. I then explained that tenderness was universally considered the hallmark of that disorder and palpation of the patient's right lower quadrant, flank, and rectum elicited no tenderness. I also noted in the record that when I palpated deep into the patient's right lower quadrant, he reported feeling better. Because the patient reported shoveling for several hours while digging a ditch (unusual work for him), described the pain as occurring in spasms, and reported relief, first with deep palpation of his abdomen and then with medication for muscle spasms, my diagnosis was abdominal wall muscle spasm.

After viewing that profile and those sources and hearing my related explanation for excluding appendicitis, the senior claims representative stated, "My gosh, your attorney will make mincemeat out of his." I never heard another word about that case. I'm still baffled by it. I may have encountered a highly unusual (reportable) presentation of appendicitis, or the disease process may have begun and rapidly progressed *after* my care. That experience, however, helped me realize the power and utility of color-assisted, Bayesian-like analysis. That claims representative told me that my ED director thought I did everything I should have done. Using the diagnostic profile and related sources convinced her of that.

CHAPTER 3

Preventing Future Burnout

THIS CHAPTER EXPLAINS how use of the HIPUS® system can prevent future burnout among physicians by optimizing use of artificial intelligence (AI) and/or machine learning (ML) clinical diagnostic products and letting physicians fully interact with those products.

Optimizing Use of AI/ML Products

Today, the use of AI/ML diagnostic products in medicine is largely limited to imaging studies (x-rays, CT scans, ultrasounds, etc.). An October 2023 US FDA listing of 692 approved AI/ML products shows use of 85 percent by radiologists, 9 percent by cardiovascular physicians/surgeons, and 1–5 percent by other specialists.[44] No products have been approved that use AI/ML to improve *clinical* diagnosis (use of symptoms, signs, and other findings to rule in or out diseases). Using the Google search engine and another provided by the National Library of Medicine (PubMed), along with various search terms, I accessed hundreds of articles covering imaging-related AI/ML products but found none covering a clinical diagnosis product that has significantly impacted care.

Imaging-related AI/ML products work well because they use the same images doctors use—in other words, the same data. A clinical diagnosis–related product won't work well or be useful enough until it uses EHR data generated via physician use of color-assisted, Bayesian-like analysis described in chapter 2. The following explains why.

From about 1970 to 1985, the US medical informatics community implemented computer-based clinical diagnostic assistance designed to replace physicians as expert diagnosticians or let them be active, information-seeking participants in the diagnostic process. They did so using data manually extracted from the medical literature or gleaned from practice experience.

As shown in the following image, none of the four systems they developed worked well enough to significantly impact medical practice.

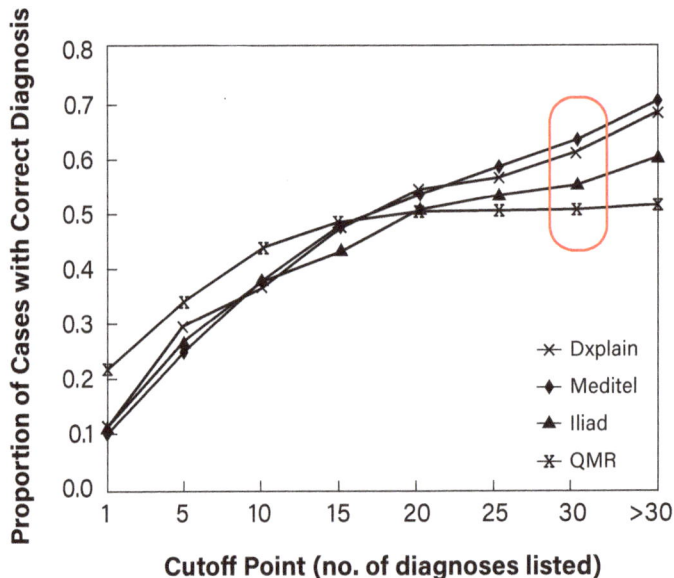

Figure 1. From 1994 NEJM article, Performance of four computer-based diagnostic systems[45]

A 1994 *The New England Journal of Medicine* article describes a study of these systems' performance.[46] As shown in this graph (included in that article) a team of thirteen MDs/PhDs found that the best one included the correct diagnosis in a list of thirty presented possibilities in less than 70 percent of cases (correct diagnosis wasn't included in more than 30 percent).

Eta Berner, EdD, who led that team, expressed great interest in the HIPUS® color-coded interface (see pioneer response, chapter 7) but also urged me to study those systems while designing mine. I therefore spent several months producing a ninety-four-page illustrated document describing the differences between the HIPUS® system and two of the previous systems—Quick Medical Reference (QMR), which models the deductive reasoning of human diagnosticians, and Iliad, one of three Bayesian systems.

I found the most important differences to be the following:

- Those systems don't facilitate the sure-footed approach to diagnosis described in chapter 2—instead of starting with one finding, the patient's chief complaint, they permit initial entry of several.

- They don't treat disease variations as separate diagnostic entities.

- They don't provide a way for physicians to readily challenge or accept a proposed diagnosis and then explain and justify doing so.

The following is an example of why starting with several findings is problematic. A patient might cite three reasons for her ED visit—fever, cough, and wheezing, suggesting airway or lung infection—when, in fact, the *main* reason is a one-day fever of 103°. The patient has had a nonproductive cough and mild wheezing for a week, which she often gets due to chronic asthma. During my practice, I found that about 95 percent of patients, if pressed, could identify a main reason, and focusing on that chief complaint helped me identify the disease requiring the most urgent or emergent care. In this example, the cause of the patient's fever might well be a serious kidney infection. The HIPUS® system allows a doctor to easily start with just one finding by giving him ways to safely limit the number of causes considered initially and know if and when others need to be considered.

The following explains the need to treat disease variations as separate diagnostic entities.

AMI: Typical	AMI: Painless	AMI: Young patient
● No troponin rise over time ** ○ Combination, H&P findings ** ●p Studies applied to low risk 　　patients ** X ECG → reperfusion therapy * 　OR X Troponin rise/fall; one value 　　> 99th percentile URL ** 　Plus additional criteria ** X Age ≥ 40 years X Pain or discomfort ** 　Pain duration > 20 minutes 　Associated signs/symptoms ** ● CAD risk factors ** 　New dysrhythmia / heart block 　Prvious MI / angina 　Other **	Same as AMI: typical ** except x Same as AMI: typical ** Anginal equivalent(s) 　Dyspnea / SOB 　Syncope or dizziness 　Weakness or fatigue 　Malaise 　Palpitations 　Vomiting 　Sweating 　Other ** Pain oblitering condition(s)... 　Age > 65 yrs 　Diabetes mellitus 　Female gender 　Others ** 　Unknown Same as AMI: typical ** except y x Pain related findings removed y Associated S/S included with 　anginl equivalents	Same as AMI: typical ** Same as AMI: typical ** except x x Age < 40 Others same as AMI: typical ** Risk factors... 　Male gender 　Cigarette smoking 　Hyperlipidemia (cholesterol) 　Family history premature CAD 　Cocaine use 　Diabetes mellitus 　Hypertension 　Systemic lupus erythematosus 　Oral contraceptive use Same as AMI: typical ** x Early repolarization with J point 　elevation occurs more often

These screens show three important variations of AMI included in the HIPUS® knowledge base—AMI: typical, AMI: painless, and AMI: young patient. Orange and yellow findings are used to rule in or out each variation—purple and green, the disease itself (all variations). After studying AMI: typical, the other variations can be easily studied by comparison. At the bedside, any can be easily selected for consideration, given need to do so, and ruling in or out any variation rules in or out the general disease.

As shown in the second screen, the presentation of AMI: painless is very different from that of AMI: typical. Presenting it as a separate entity for study and bedside use helps the physician to not overlook the diagnosis of AMI. Presenting AMI: young patient separately lets the physician focus on important related info: (1) A largely benign ECG pattern that closely resembles a heart attack pattern is much more often present with young patients and easily prompts needless, costly, and/or risky additional care; and (2) risk factors are generally more important and different in young patients, especially women.

Other HIPUS® knowledge base disease variations include:

PULMONARY EMBOLISM	PNEUMOTHORAX	PNEUMONIA
PE: with collapse (massive)	PT: tension	PN: community acquired
PE: isolated	PT: primary spontaneous	PN: hospital acquired/ ventilator associated
PE: superimposed (comorbidity)	PT: secondary spontaneous (comorbidity)	

As with AMI, the HIPUS® system uses a handful of orange and/or yellow findings to clearly characterize each disease variation (distinguish it from others). Presenting all of those findings in one "profile" would be more confusing than helpful and would *not* clearly characterize the general disease. That might be another reason the four systems previously described often failed to identify and present the correct diagnosis within a list of possibilities.

Not allowing physicians to readily challenge or accept a proposed diagnosis and then explain and justify doing so makes diagnostic assistance not very useful. By converting alphanumeric data indicating finding specificity/sensitivity, easily processed by computers, to color-coded data, easily processed by humans, the HIPUS® system can effectively address that problem.

Again, since those four systems were built, no other system providing computer-based clinical diagnostic assistance has impacted care enough to be viable. Furthermore, the way diagnostic information is presented to and used by physicians hasn't changed enough to permit the creation of viable assistance—certainly not enough to permit the color-assisted, Bayesian-like analysis described in chapter 2.

Dr. Carol Rivers strongly endorsed not only the HIPUS® color-coded interface but also the knowledge base I constructed for heart attack variations. Using an expanded version of that knowledge base when generating EHRs will provide data needed to create a viable AI/ML product.

The following explains how that might be done.

Articles published in 2017 and 2020 describe and then evaluate the combined use of diagnostic data extracted from 270,000 ED records (EHRs) and various ML algorithms to produce knowledge graphs that establish statistically significant relationships or edges between diseases and symptoms.[47, 48] I created the following figure to show a simple example of such a knowledge graph.

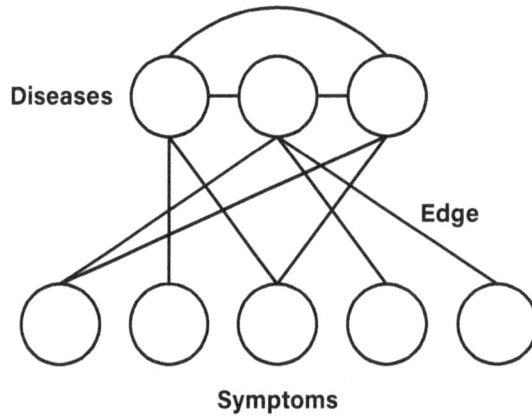

Figure 2. Author-created example of a knowledge graph.

A Google Health Knowledge Graph (GHKG), manually created by physicians, was used to determine which diseases and symptoms to extract from those EHRs. The authors of the first article then tested use of different ML algorithms to determine which produced a knowledge graph that best resembled the GHKG.

The pioneering effort described and discussed in those articles is an essential first step toward implementing ED use of a viable AI/ML diagnostic product. The methodology is certainly much better than that used fifty years ago, but data provided by current EHRs doesn't permit use of that methodology to provide fully functional diagnostic assistance. EHRs generated via physician use of color-assisted, Bayesian-like analysis can let a modified and expanded version of the ML product produced by that effort determine the most likely cause of a patient's chief complaint by using not just diseases but also clearly established and defined disease variations, and not just symptoms but also other findings—symptoms, signs, test results and other factors. Furthermore, it can use the specificity and/or sensitivity of each finding for each disease variation, determined via medical literature search and analysis.

As explained in several articles, to be fully functional, an AI/ML product must use not only all needed data but also high-quality data.[49, 50, 51]

The authors of a 2022 article state: "Until recently, both academia and industry were mainly engaged in introducing new or improving existing machine learning (ML) models, rather than finding remedies for any data challenges that fall beyond trivial cleaning or preparation steps. Nevertheless, the performance of AI-enhanced systems in practice is proven to be bounded by the quality of the underlying training data."[52]

Those articles discuss common criteria used to measure data quality, including the following:

- Accuracy: Does the data reflect the real-world object and/or events it is intended to model? Accuracy is partly assessed by the extent to which the data is provided using credible information sources—for example, reputable medical textbooks and peer-reviewed journal articles.

- Completeness: Does the data contain all required records and values? Completeness of data ensures that an AI/ML product has all the information needed to provide quality analysis—for example, info provided via use of color-assisted, Bayesian-like analysis.

- Granularity: Does the data describe the patient's condition with sufficient detail to permit quality analysis? For example, does it contain all checklist finding entries needed to rule in or out any considered disease variation using corresponding profile findings?

- Consistency: Is all similar data presented using the same data format or structure? Such consistency is needed to permit effective data integration and includes consistent use of related definitions and codes—for example, those provided by the Unified Medical Language System and ICD-10 codes.

- Timeliness: Is the data updated frequently or in real time to permit the best use of AI/ML products? Most medical data needs to be updated *at least* once a year.

- Validity: Does the data conform to established business (or medical practice) rules and meet allowable parameters? Validity helps ensure that the data can be used to perform certain tasks—for example, providing patient data for bedside assistance without violating HIPAA regulations, which protect patient privacy.

As described in chapter 2, when a physician uses the HIPUS® system to perform color-assisted, Bayesian-like analysis, the vast majority of data used will be extracted from a relational database (RDB) and downloaded to a mobile device for use by its applications. The HIPUS® RDB has been meticulously designed to produce and maintain data quality that meets these six and other criteria.

Letting Physicians Fully Interact with AI/ML Products

Documenting use of that data within EHRs will let a modified version of the aforementioned ML product use the same data physicians use. When a concluded diagnosis is presented, the HIPUS® system can convert alphanumeric indicators of finding specificity and/or sensitivity for each diagnosis variation to colored indicators used by physicians and thereby permit seamless doctor–product collaboration. Also, the product can learn from physician challenges or input to improve diagnostic assistance in the future.

Physicians will need to construct the initial HIPUS® knowledge base. After that task has been completed, however, the vast majority of knowledge base work will involve updating its content. Large Language Models (LLMs) can let physicians perform that task with much greater ease and speed. LLMs that can do so are more sophisticated versions of Chat GPT, which understands and generates humanlike text when performing simpler tasks. LLM-related technology is rapidly improving in two ways:

- The models themselves are getting better.

- The prompts needed to elicit useful and accurate LLM responses are also improving due to advancements in the field of prompt engineering.

The following describes how I used the model GPT-4o to update a small part of the knowledge base for AMI: typical, constructed in 2021

I chose to update the following part:

3 X New or presumed new LBBB

New or presumed new left bundle branch block (LBBB) is presented as an indication for reperfusion therapy in the 2020 *ACLS Provider Manual* and 2018 expert consensus document, "Fourth Universal Definition of Myocardial Infarction."[i, ii] The latter states: "Comparison to a pre-admission ECG may be helpful in determining if the conduction defect or ST-T wave changes are new, as long as it does not delay time to treatment. Ischemic symptoms and presumed new LBBB that is not rate-related are associated with an adverse prognosis."[ii]

i.   American Heart Association. *Advanced Cardiac Life Support Provider Manual*. American Heart Association; 2020.

ii. Thygesen K, Alpert JS, Jaffe AS, et al.; Executive Group on behalf of the Joint ESC/ACCF/AHA/WHF Task Force for the Universal Definition of Myocardial Infarction. Fourth universal definition of myocardial infarction. *Circulation*. 2018 Nov 13;138(20): e618-e651. doi:10.1161/CIR.0000000000000617

To update the knowledge base, I first conducted a National Library of Medicine PubMed search using the terms or keywords "diagnosis," "acute myocardial infarction," and "left bundle branch block" to look for related journal articles I might have overlooked when producing the prior statements or any articles published more recently. I found six such articles:

i.   Nestelberger T, Cullen L, Lindahl B, et al. Diagnosis of acute myocardial infarction in the presence of left bundle branch block. *Heart*. 2019 Oct;105(20):1559-1567. doi:10.1136/heartjnl-2018-314673

ii.   Di Marco A, Rodriguez M, Cinca J, et al. New electrocardiographic algorithm for the diagnosis of acute myocardial infarction in patients with left bundle branch block. *J Am Heart Assoc*. 2020 Jul 21;9(14):e015573. doi:10.1161/JAHA.119.015573

iii. Lai Y, Chen Y-H, Wu K-H, Chen Y-C. Validation of the diagnosis and triage algorithm for acute myocardial infarction in the setting of left bundle branch block. *Am J Emerg Med*. 2020 Dec;38(12):2614-2619. doi:10.1016/j.ajem.2020.03.024

iv.   Macfarlane PW. New ECG criteria for acute myocardial infarction in patients with left bundle branch block. *J Am Heart Assoc*. 2020 Jul 21;9(14):e017119. doi:10.1161/JAHA.120.017119

v.   Nestelberger T, Boeddinghaus J, Lopez Ayala P, et al. Utility of echocardiography in patients with suspected acute myocardial infarction and left bundle-branch block. *J Am Heart Assoc*. 2021 Sep 21;10(18):e021262. doi:10.1161/JAHA.121.021262

vi.   Friesinger GC, Smith RF. Old age, left bundle branch block and acute myocardial infarction: a vexing and lethal combination. *J Am Coll Cardiol*. 2000;36:713-716. doi:10.1016/s0735-1097(00)00801-9

Via the OpenAI API, built and made available by the makers of ChatGPT, I then checked to see if those articles contained any information that might be used to update that HIPUS® knowledge base part. To do so, I used an updating assistant created by a data scientist with abundant related expertise. That assistant provided general instructions for use by *any* LLM, specified which model would be used (GPT-4o) and how, and permitted user entry of a specific prompt covering use of *vectorized* statements and articles. How that text is vectorized is described later in this chapter.

The GPT-4o model found such information in three of those articles—1, 2, and 4—and used it to suggest updates. I then used those suggested updates, in this case verbatim, to modify the HIPUS® knowledge base part as shown in the last two paragraphs. I also added citations (iii–v) of the articles used by that model to produce those suggested updates.

3 X New or presumed new LBBB

New or presumed new LBBB is presented as an indication for reperfusion therapy in the 2020 ACLS Provider Manual and expert consensus document, Fourth Universal Definition of Myocardial Infarction.[i, ii] The latter states: "Comparison to a pre-admission ECG may be helpful in determining if the conduction defect or ST-T wave changes are new, as long as it does not delay time to treatment. Ischemic symptoms and presumed new LBBB that is not rate-related are associated with an adverse prognosis."[ii]

However, combining ECG criteria with high-sensitivity cardiac troponin (hs-cTnT/I) testing at one hour or two hours allows for early and accurate diagnosis of AMI in patients with LBBB. This combined approach has shown high diagnostic accuracy, with an area under the ROC curve (AUC) of 0.91 for hs-cTnT and 0.89 for hs-cTnI.[iii]

Recent studies have also introduced new criteria for diagnosing AMI in patients with LBBB. The new Barcelona algorithm, which includes criteria, such as ST depression ≥0.1 mV in any lead where the QRS complex is concordant and ST deviation ≥0.1 mV in any lead where the dominant QRS wave is ≤0.6 mV, has shown high sensitivity (93 percent) and specificity (94 percent).[iv, v]

i. American Heart Association. *Advanced Cardiac Life Support Provider Manual.* American Heart Association; 2020.

ii.   Thygesen K, Alpert JS, Jaffe AS, et al.; Executive Group on behalf of the Joint ESC/ACCF/AHA/WHF Task Force for the Universal Definition of Myocardial Infarction. Fourth universal definition of myocardial infarction. *Circulation*. 2018 Nov 13;138(20). doi:10.1161/CIR.0000000000000617

iii. Nestelberger T, et al. Diagnosis of acute myocardial infarction in the presence of left bundle branch block. Heart. 2019 Oct;105(20):1559-1567.

iv.   Di Marco A, et al. New Electrocardiographic Algorithm for the Diagnosis of Acute Myocardial Infarction in Patients With Left Bundle Branch Block**.** J Am Heart Assoc. 2020 Jul 21;9(14):e015573.

v.   Macfarlane PW. New ECG Criteria for Acute Myocardial Infarction in Patients With Left Bundle Branch Block. J Am Heart Assoc. 2020 Jul 21; 9(14): e017119.

The following describes how the entire HIPUS® knowledge base might be updated with greater ease and speed using the OpenAI API or a similar platform.

The OpenAI API permits use of vector stores containing up to ten thousand articles. Pinecone Systems, Inc., creator of the first vector store, offers a product that stores more than a million. All PubMed articles published after a certain date might be stored in one or the other.

An LLM such as Med-PaLM, specifically designed for use in medicine, might be employed to process the text in those articles.

Rather than using the PubMed search engine and search terms or keywords, that model could use vectorized articles to better identify those related to each vectorized statement. Unlike keyword-based searches that rely on exact matches, vectorization allows the system to understand the context and meaning behind words, leading to more accurate and comprehensive search results.

The following is a simple example of how text might be vectorized.

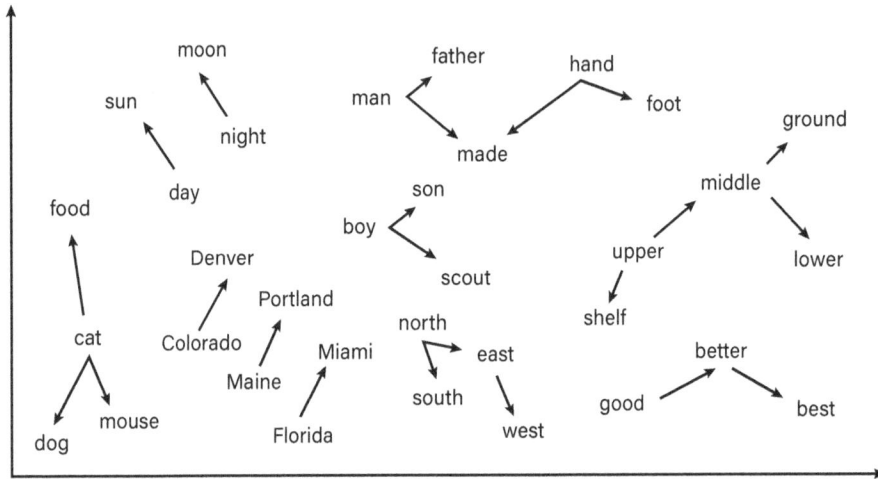

Figure 3. Author-created example of vectorized text, based on a similar example in
Generative AI and LLMs For Dummies.[53]

Each word is related to one or more other words that are frequently used with it. Each word is represented by a number in a multidimensional space. Use of such vector "embeddings" is the most efficient way to store and process quantitative representations of natural language. Useful data (text) can be identified based on similarity metrics, such as distance between two vectors, instead of exact matches, which saves a tremendous amount of processing time and greatly improves use of natural language. A selected LLM (Med-PaLM) can use vectorized text in each HIPUS® knowledge base statement and the articles to present update suggestions along with supporting source (article) citations. Use of those suggestions to modify each knowledge base part might also be automated.

Physicians will always need to check and perhaps edit suggested updates, but use of this process to update the entire HIPUS® knowledge base can dramatically reduce the human time and effort needed to do so.

CHAPTER 4

Improving Doctor–Nurse Collaboration

AS MUCH AS I DISLIKED nurse interference with my practice, I've come to understand it. Conversing with ED nurses helped me realize that having to execute orders generated by physicians who often seem, or clearly are, incompetent, and having little or no power to influence such care, is demoralizing to them. While not yet fully addressed by the current EM certification process, this problem was likely worse before that process was established in 1980 and fully implemented over the next several years. Older nurses who are now supervisors bore the brunt of the problem. Furthermore, nurses can't easily avoid working with doctors who provide poor care, which likely prompted some to control or displace physician practice with a vengeance.

On the other hand, some of my best memories of EM practice involve successful collaboration with nurses. Examples include those that made possible or produced

- successful immediate pericardiocentesis, never performed before by any of us—nurses immediately provided exactly what was needed;

- successful, simultaneous management of a patient with a ruptured spleen and another in the middle of a complicated psychiatric crisis; and

- unusually detailed nurse documentation of circumstances related to the physical restraint of a patient, which perfectly complemented mine and fully explained the need for such restraint.

The 2015 IOM report *Improving Diagnosis in Health Care* discusses the importance of diagnosis-related collaboration. It begins by stating: "Nurses can play a key role in the diagnostic process. They therefore need to be full and active members of the diagnostic team, with opportunities to present their observations and conclusions to other team members."[54]

A related 2021 article in *Nursing Outlook*, the official journal of the American Academy of Nursing and the Council for the Advancement of Nursing Science, wholly endorses that IOM report's call for such collaboration and discusses educational steps needed to achieve it. The authors conclude: "To better serve our patients, the diagnostic process must improve. Nurses are in an ideal position to play a central role in achieving diagnostic excellence…. Yet, many nurses enter practice with an antiquated belief that diagnosis is not in their domain, and they are not prepared to participate in the process. It is crucial for nursing education to address this misperception, and [prepare nurses to be] participants on the diagnostic team."[55]

That 2015 IOM report suggests several ways nurses might participate in and thereby improve diagnosis, including:

- knowing the major diagnoses of patients;

- being the eyes of the diagnostic team by detecting, reporting, and documenting changes in patients' symptoms, signs, complaints, or conditions;

- helping optimize communication between patients and the care teams by helping patients tell their story and report all of their symptoms and checking patients' understanding of their diagnoses and what they've been told;

- learning about how diagnostic errors arise and how they can be avoided;

- educating patients about the diagnostic process;

- educating patients about diagnostic tests and explaining why they are needed, what the patient will experience, and what the results will reveal; and

- helping patients with the emotional and psychological difficulties that arise when a diagnosis is not yet known or is known to be bad.[56]

> *The HIPUS® knowledge base will provide a solid basis for such collaboration. Color-assisted, Bayesian-like analysis will permit doctor–nurse use of that knowledge base in the best possible way.*

The slideshow "Nurse Care" at hipus.care was created *as a first step* toward improving such collaboration. It shows how a nurse might use a mobile device and applications, similar to those designed for doctors, to perform nursing tasks.

The following is intended as a supplement to that slideshow. It presents examples of how a nurse might use that device and those applications to view info being used by the doctor, see *how* it's being used throughout the diagnostic process, and participate in ways called for in the aforementioned IOM report.

The following screens show the main menus a nurse might use (the same as those shown in the "Nurse Care" slideshow).

Routine Care	⌖ SORT			
PATIENT INFO: 8	LOCATION	TESTS		
Fever	⌖ 4	~		
3 YR M • Coleman, Eric	1:59 AM			
Chest Pain	⌖ C2	○		
64 YR M • John Bradford	1:45 AM			
Abd Pain	⌖ 2	⊘		
58 YR F • Kroeger, Gladys	12:20 AM			
Rash	⌖ 8	~		
9 MO F • Faircloth, Susan	11:52 PM			
SOB	⌖ C1	⊙		
65 YR F • Miller, Ruth	11:38 PM			
Ankle Injury	⌖ CR	⊘		
14 YR M • Hinesman, John	9:45 PM			
Headache	⌖ 6	~		
40 YR F • Chaffier, Lois	9:03 PM			
Depression	⌖ Psy	○		
52 YR M • Mckinley, Chad	8:42 PM			

Bradford, John

Chest pain • 64 YR M • 2:05 AM ⌖ C2

i O A

Execute orders

Established by protocol

Generated by physician

Access related care info

Bradford, John

Chest pain • 64 YR M • 2:05 AM ⌖ C2

i O A

Assess response to care

Address other patient problems or requests

Access related care info

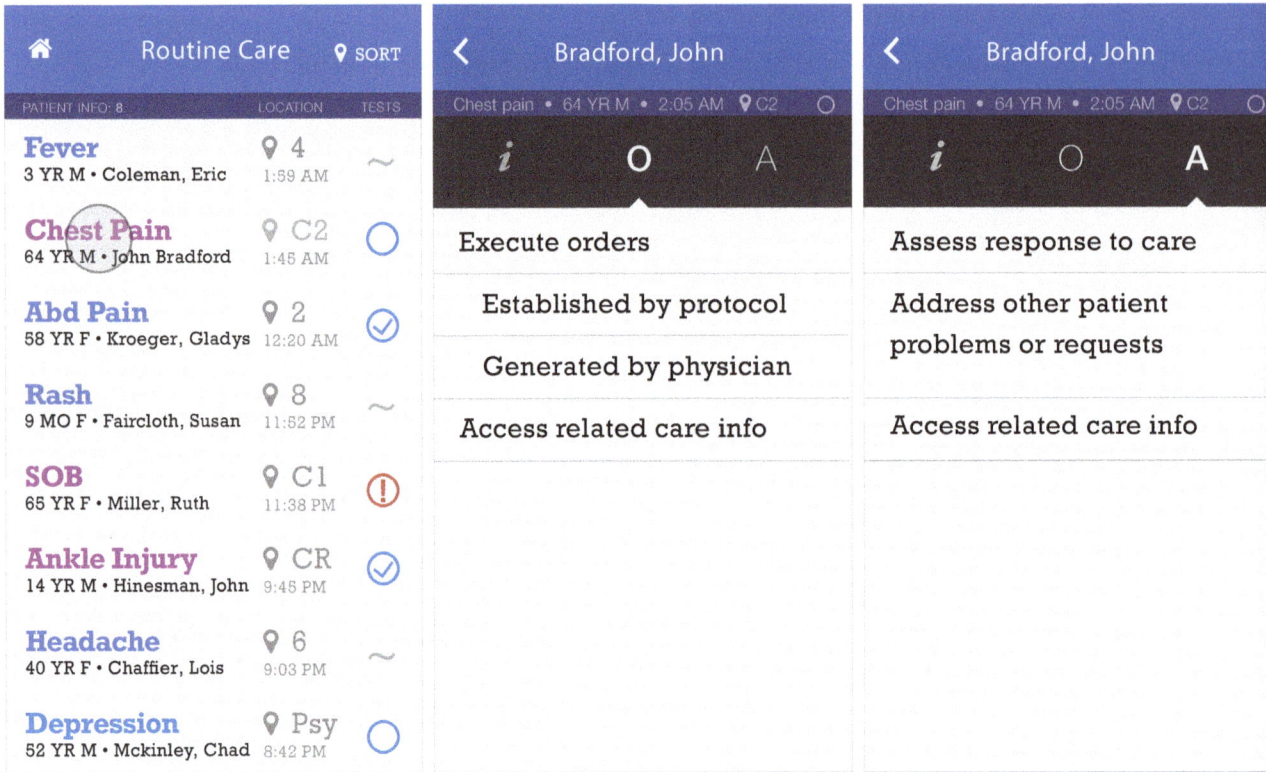

Note: Immediate care menus, not shown here, will also be included in nurse applications.

The Routine Care menu is essentially the same as that used by the doctor, except that purple indicates patients being cared for primarily by the nurse. The orders (O) and assessment (A) menus are used to provide, document, and report care. The last item on both lets a nurse access info being used or generated by the doctor to perform those tasks. The following pages present examples of how a nurse might use that info to participate in and improve diagnosis. To simplify gender use, in each example the doctor is a female—the nurse, a male.

Bradford, John

Chest pain • 64 YR M • 2:05 AM • C2

i   ○   **A**

Assess response to care

Address other patient problems or requests

Access related care info

Bradford, John

Related care information

MIP: Chest pain

Diagnosis …

  Dxs being considered …

    Emergent **

    Non-emergent **

  Dxs not being considered **

  Dx concluded

Treatment **

Disposition **

Bradford, John

Related care information

MIP: Chest pain

Diagnosis …

  Dxs being considered …

    Emergent …

    AMI: typical

    Unstable angina

    Aortic dissection: typical

  Non-emergent **

  Dxs not being considered **

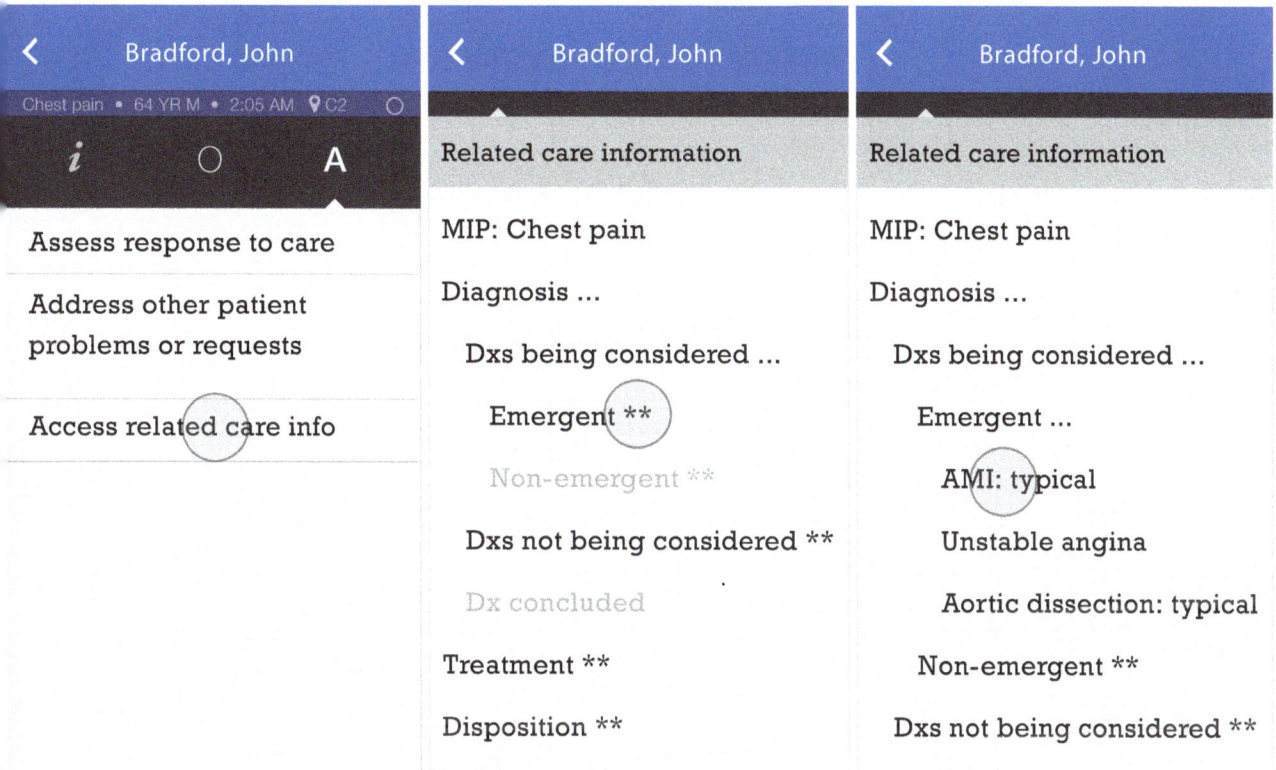

After tapping on the last menu item on the first screen, the nurse makes a series of choices (next screen), which lets him see which emergent diseases (those requiring hospitalization) are being considered. In this case, as seen on the last screen, they are AMI, UA, and aortic dissection. Aortic dissection is tearing of the inner aortic wall within the chest, permitting blood to fill the space between wall layers and/or penetrate the outer layer and spill into the chest cavity—the latter being fatal. Disease variations are treated as separate diagnostic entities. AMI: typical is heart attack with typical symptoms in patients more than forty years old. Aortic dissection: typical is acute (versus chronic) dissection in patients more than forty years old. Tapping on "AMI: typical" …

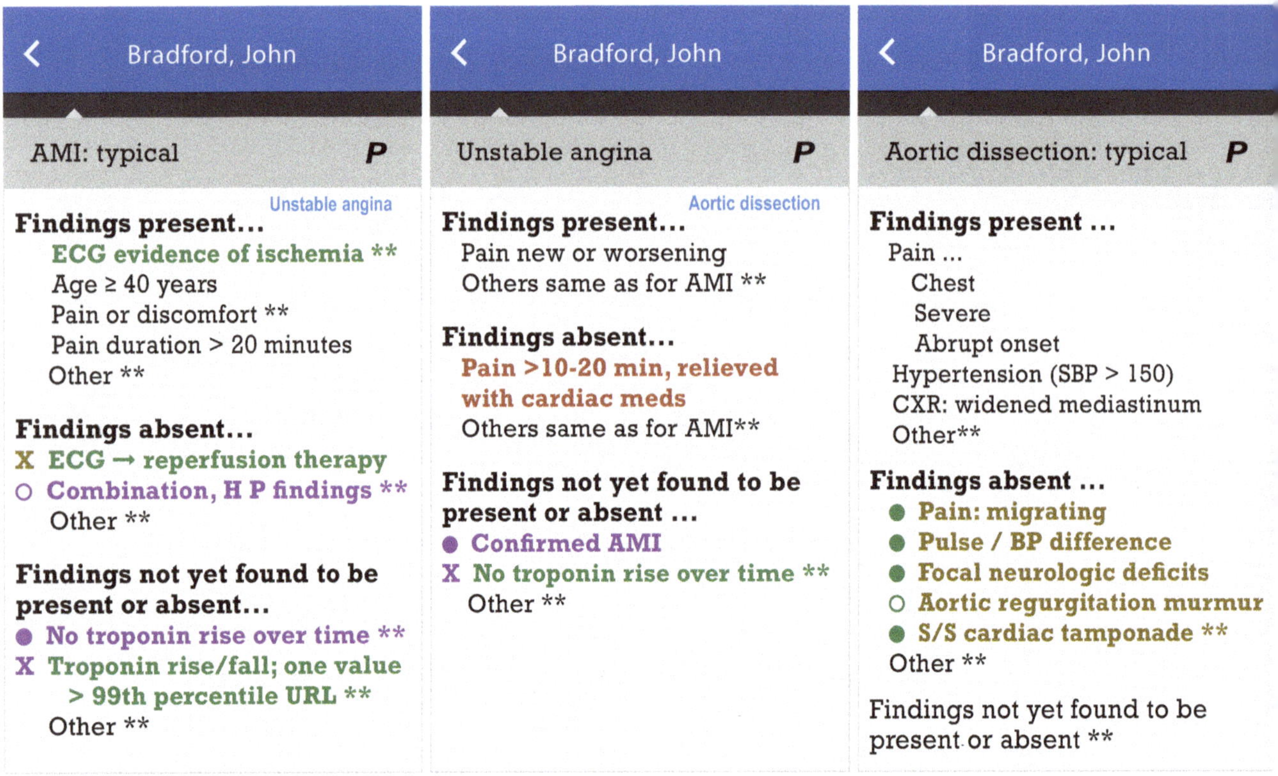

‹ Bradford, John

AMI: typical   **P**

Unstable angina

Findings present...
  ECG evidence of ischemia **
  Age ≥ 40 years
  Pain or discomfort **
  Pain duration > 20 minutes
  Other **

Findings absent...
X **ECG → reperfusion therapy**
O **Combination, H P findings **
  Other **

**Findings not yet found to be
present or absent...**
● **No troponin rise over time **
X **Troponin rise/fall; one value
   > 99th percentile URL **
  Other **

‹ Bradford, John

Unstable angina   **P**

Aortic dissection

Findings present...
  Pain new or worsening
  Others same as for AMI **

Findings absent...
  **Pain >10-20 min, relieved
  with cardiac meds**
  Others same as for AMI**

**Findings not yet found to be
present or absent ...**
● **Confirmed AMI**
X **No troponin rise over time **
  Other **

‹ Bradford, John

Aortic dissection: typical   **P**

Findings present ...
  Pain ...
    Chest
    Severe
    Abrupt onset
  Hypertension (SBP > 150)
  CXR: widened mediastinum
  Other**

Findings absent ...
● **Pain: migrating**
● **Pulse / BP difference**
● **Focal neurologic deficits**
O **Aortic regurgitation murmur**
● **S/S cardiac tamponade **
  Other **

Findings not yet found to be
present or absent **

… lets the nurse view the first screen shown here. Tapping on "Unstable angina" (right upper corner of the first screen) and "Aortic dissection" (next screen) lets him view the last two. How these screens might be used by nurses is described later in this chapter.

These screens were produced by the system in response to physician use of checklist findings and the Bayesian menu described in chapter 2. In this case, however, the diagnosis has *not* yet been concluded. The info presented is periodically updated as the doctor works toward a diagnosis.

The patient, John Bradford, a sixty-four-year-old with a history of AMI, presents with a chief complaint of severe chest pain, which began abruptly twenty minutes prior to his ED arrival at 1:45 a.m. The physician takes a brief history, performs a physical exam, and views the ECG and bedside chest x-ray. Routine lab test results, including a blood troponin level (indicator of heart damage), are not yet available.

Mr. Bradford's pain is not relieved by meds that usually relieve anginal (heart) pain. His blood pressure is 185/100 and his heart rate is 124 (both seriously elevated). His ECG indicates ischemia (poor oxygen supply) but not a heart attack or need for reperfusion (blood clot removing) therapy. His chest x-ray is otherwise normal, but the physician thinks it might show a widened mediastinum (portion of the chest containing the aorta)—a sign of possible aortic dissection.

Given Mr. Bradford's history of AMI and current ECG pattern, the physician chooses to consider AMI and UA. But given his report of sudden, severe pain and what may be a widened mediastinum, she also considers aortic dissection a real possibility requiring her immediate attention. After reducing the patient's pain and blood pressure (using different meds), the doctor works through related checklist findings and considers the implications of her entries via the Bayesian menu. The system then allows the nurse to access related info shown in the following images.

< Bradford, John

AMI: typical **P**

Unstable angina

Findings present...
  ECG evidence of ischemia **
  Age ≥ 40 years
  Pain or discomfort **
  Pain duration > 20 minutes
  Other **

Findings absent...
X **ECG → reperfusion therapy**
O **Combination, H P findings ****
  Other **

Findings not yet found to be present or absent...
● **No troponin rise over time ****
X **Troponin rise/fall; one value > 99th percentile URL ****
  Other **

< Bradford, John

Unstable angina **P**

Aortic dissection

Findings present...
  Pain new or worsening
  Others same as for AMI **

Findings absent...
  Pain >10-20 min, relieved with cardiac meds
  Others same as for AMI**

Findings not yet found to be present or absent ...
● **Confirmed AMI**
X **No troponin rise over time ****
  Other **

< Bradford, John

Aortic dissection: typical **P**

Findings present ...
  Pain ...
    Chest
    Severe
    Abrupt onset
  Hypertension (SBP > 150)
  CXR: widened mediastinum
  Other**

Findings absent ...
● **Pain: migrating**
● **Pulse / BP difference**
● **Focal neurologic deficits**
O **Aortic regurgitation murmur**
● **S/S cardiac tamponade ****
  Other **

Findings not yet found to be present or absent **

The main things to know about these screens are:

To present a useful but not overwhelming amount of info, the system initially presents the most useful (most sensitive or specific) findings and allows a nurse to access less useful findings by tapping on "Other." Generally, the most useful are purple, green, and orange. See color scheme on page 2.

Most findings found to be present on each screen are orange profile findings. Again, they're presented here using black font because orange indicates sensitivity or frequency of occurrence. When orange findings are *present*, their frequency of occurrence is irrelevant. One finding found to be *absent* is presented using orange font because its sensitivity *is* relevant.

Generally, the presence or absence of yellow findings is least helpful. Several yellow findings for aortic dissection, however, while not sensitive, are quite specific for that disorder (the presence of any makes aortic dissection more or much more likely). Hence, each has a green circle or dot as a secondary color. See secondary colors on page 2.

Bradford, John   <

AMI: typical   (**P**)

Unstable angina

Findings present...
   ECG evidence of ischemia *
   Age ≥ 40 years
   Pain or discomfort **
   Pain duration > 20 minutes
   Other **

Findings absent...
X **ECG → reperfusion therapy**
O **Combination, H P findings ***
   Other **

Findings not yet found to be present or absent...
● **No troponin rise over time ***
X **Troponin rise/fall; one value > 99th percentile URL ***
   Other **

Bradford, John   <

AMI: typical profile   ✔

● **No troponin rise over time ***
O **Combination, H&P findings ***
●ₚ **Studies applied to low risk patients ***

X **ECG → reperfusion therapy ***
OR
X **Troponin rise/fall; one value > 99th percentile URL ***
   Plus additional criteria *

X **Age ≥ 40 years**
X **Pain or discomfort ***
   Pain duration > 20 minutes

   Associated signs/symptoms *
● **CAD risk factors ***
   Other *

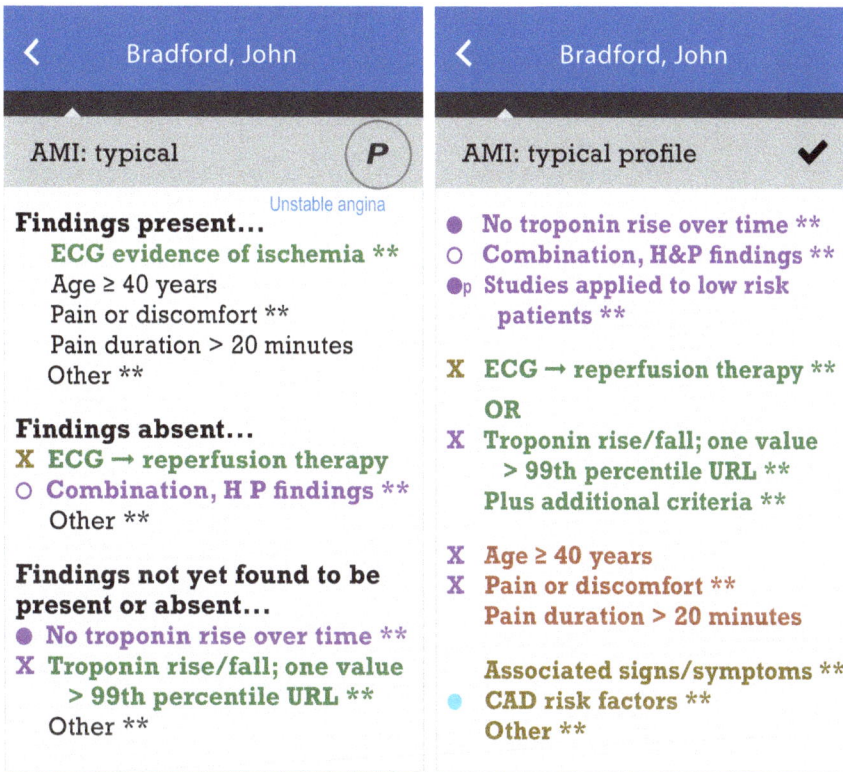

At any time while viewing any of the previous screens, by tapping on the profile icon (*P*), a nurse can view the diagnostic profile for that disease (all findings that might be used to rule it in or out) and then, by tapping on the checklist icon (✔), return to that screen to see which findings have and haven't been used.

Nurses can learn to understand and use all these screens fairly quickly.

The following pages present examples of how a nurse might use info in these and other screens to improve diagnosis-related care per IOM recommendations.

The following shows how a nurse might be the eyes of the diagnostic team by detecting and reporting changes in patient symptoms, signs, complaints, or conditions.

In this case, the best available way to rule in or out aortic dissection is by performing a contrast enhanced helical CT imaging study (a sophisticated CT scan using contrast material). Before calling in a radiologist and giving the on-call surgeon a heads-up, the physician hopes to obtain more evidence supporting that diagnosis.

Bradford, John <

Aortic dissection: typical   *P*

Findings present …
Pain …
  Chest
  Severe
  Abrupt onset
Hypertension (SBP > 150)
CXR: widened mediastinum
Other**

Findings absent …
● **Pain: migrating**
● **Pulse / BP difference**
● **Focal neurologic deficits**
○ **Aortic regurgitation murmur**
● **S/S cardiac tamponade ***
Other **

Findings not yet found to be present or absent **

Any of these yellow findings not present initially might become so as blood between the aortic wall layers advances in either direction and thereby (1) causes the pain to migrate; (2) blocks flow to branching arteries, producing a weak pulse in one arm or causing parts of the nervous system to shut down; (3) damages the aortic valve; and/or (4) fills the sac around the heart, preventing it from expanding enough to pump needed blood.

While the doctor's time and attention are consumed by caring for patients with acute, severe abdominal pain and shortness of breath, the nurse uses that list of yellow findings to periodically check for the presence of any of them. By doing so, he finds that the patient's pain has migrated—it is now present in his chest *and* neck—and that the patient's blood pressure in his right arm is 82/50 mmHg, compared to 145/85 in his left arm. The nurse then reports that to the physician who, after confirming both, uses the Bayesian menu to indicate the presence of those findings. The physician then asks the on-call radiologist to perform a helical CT scan and discusses the patient's likely diagnosis with the surgeon.

The following shows how a nurse might optimize doctor–patient communication by addressing patient anxiety.

After the physician has explained why she considers a heart attack or unstable angina unlikely, both can only be ruled in or out using a series of blood tests over time, and a CT scan must be used as soon as possible to rule in or out aortic dissection, the nurse first addresses Mr. Bradford's and his wife's anxiety by answering their questions regarding the likely outcome given aortic dissection.

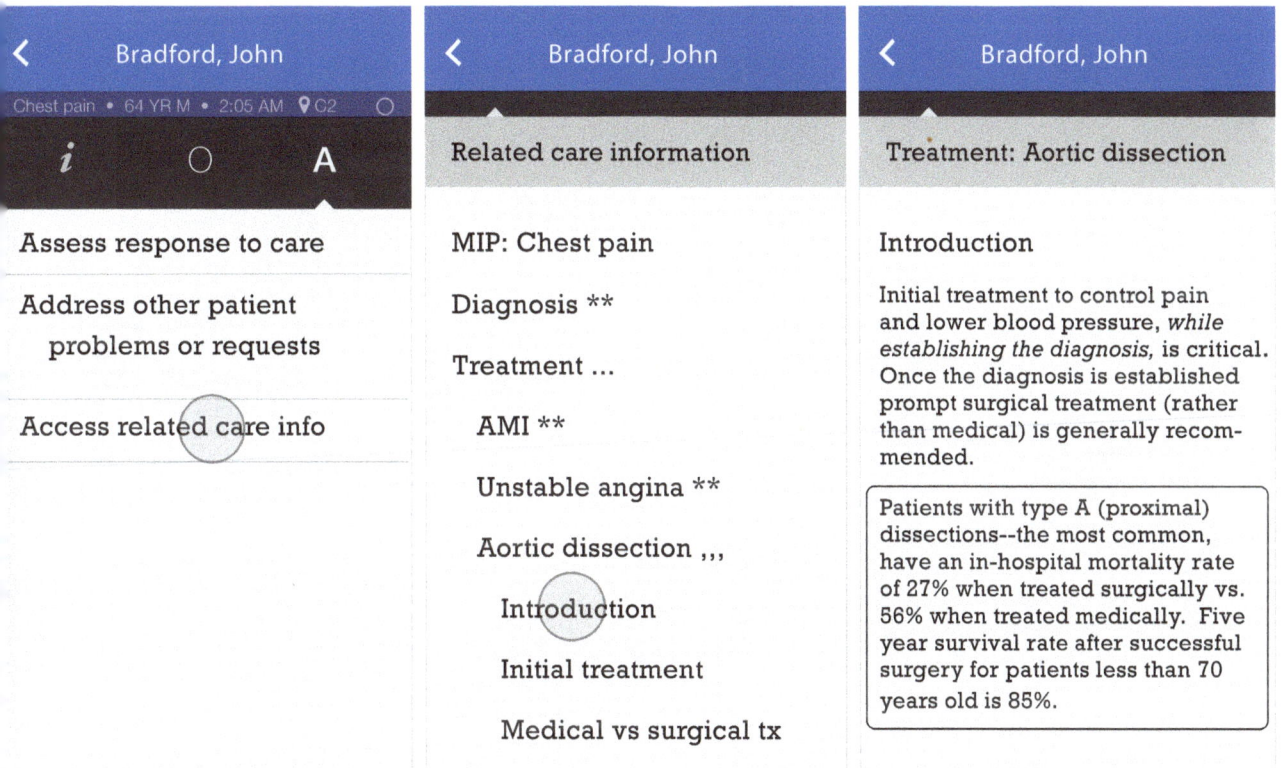

‹ Bradford, John	‹ Bradford, John	‹ Bradford, John
Chest pain • 64 YR M • 2:05 AM ♀ C2 ○		
i ○ **A**	Related care information	Treatment: Aortic dissection
Assess response to care	MIP: Chest pain	Introduction
Address other patient problems or requests	Diagnosis **	Initial treatment to control pain and lower blood pressure, *while establishing the diagnosis,* is critical. Once the diagnosis is established prompt surgical treatment (rather than medical) is generally recommended.
Access related care info	Treatment ...	
	AMI **	Patients with type A (proximal) dissections--the most common, have an in-hospital mortality rate of 27% when treated surgically vs. 56% when treated medically. Five year survival rate after successful surgery for patients less than 70 years old is 85%.
	Unstable angina **	
	Aortic dissection ,,,	
	Introduction	
	Initial treatment	
	Medical vs surgical tx	

The nurse does so by reviewing what he learned while caring for a patient with dissection nine months earlier. He accesses the related knowledge base segment by tapping on the last menu item on the first screen, making a series of choices using the second screen and viewing aortic dissection treatment info on the third (treatment info usually covers all variations of each disease). He then discusses what he recalls with Mr. and Mrs. Bradford regarding the relatively good in-hospital and five-year survival rates after prompt surgery for the most common type of aortic dissection in patients less than seventy years old.

The following shows how a nurse might discuss the ordered helical CT imaging study.

After using the first (updated) screen to explain why aortic dissection is the most likely diagnosis, the nurse addresses Mr. and Mrs. Bradford's questions about the test ordered to help rule out or confirm that diagnosis.

< Bradford, John	< Bradford, John	< Bradford, John
Aortic dissection: typical **P**	Aortic dissection: typical **P**	Aortic dissection: typical **P**

Screen 1:

Findings present ...
 Pain ...
  Chest
  Severe
  Abrupt onset
 Hypertension (SBP > 150)
● Pain migration
● Pulse / BP difference
 CXR: widened mediastinum
 Other**

Findings absent ...
● **Focal neurologic deficits**
○ **Aortic regurgitation murmur**
● **S/S cardiac tamponade **
 Other **

Findings not yet found to be present or absent **

Screen 2:

Findings not yet found to be present or absent ...

Negative imaging study ...
● MDCT
○ Helical CT
○ TEE
○ MRI

Positive imaging study ...
X MDCT
X Helical CT
X TEE
X TTE
X MRI

Screen 3:

○ **Negative imaging study: Helical CT**

Presence makes diagnosos unlikely: sensigtivity is nearly, but not 100%

Contrast enhanced Helical CT is highly sensitive for aortic dissection, but not 100%. If MDCT is not available it is anacceptable alternative. However, given high clinical suspicion for AD, a negative study is an indication for a different imaging study.

Risks include possible contrast reaction, potential for decompensation outside the ED, and ionizing radiation exposure. A relative contraindication is impaired renal function.

He does that by tapping on the double asterisk (first screen), which shows him findings that might be present or absent given the use of related imaging studies (second screen). Tapping on the purple "Helical CT" lets the nurse view statements about that study (last screen). Tapping on the green "Helical CT" lets him view similar info (not shown). The nurse then discusses that test with Mr. and Mrs. Bradford, answers related questions, and double-checks for any contraindications.

On the last screen, tapping on the purple circle presented the meaning of that secondary color—in two parts. The first part, presented using purple font, is always the same for that symbol, which helps users memorize the meaning of that symbol over time. The second part, presented using black font, provides disease (aortic dissection)-specific info.

The following shows how a nurse might prompt consideration of a diagnosis initially overlooked.

The physician is in the middle of an unusually busy and stressful shift due to an ice storm that began twelve hours earlier. By eleven o'clock that morning, she's already seen twenty-one patients. Michelle Davis, a thirty-year-old patient, complains of left, lower, anterior chest pain, which began after she slipped and fell, landing on her left side. The physician, after viewing Michelle's normal chest x-ray and finding tenderness but no contusion or abrasion on physical exam, considers simple chest wall contusion a possibility but is not sure, and she must care for a newly arrived patient with a stroke requiring immediate reperfusion therapy. The physician therefore asks the nurse to review disorders not yet considered and let her know if any seem more likely.

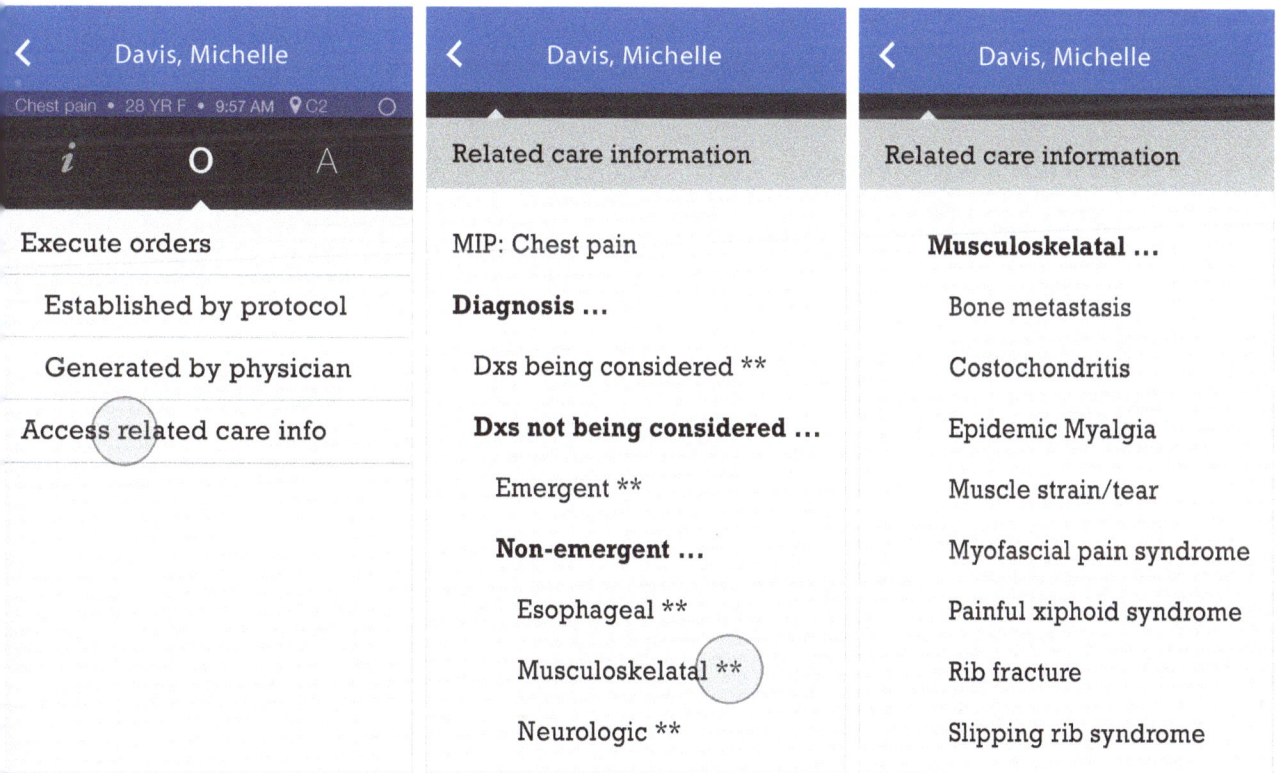

Davis, Michelle	Davis, Michelle	Davis, Michelle
Chest pain • 28 YR F • 9:57 AM ♀ C2	Related care information	Related care information
_i_ O A		
Execute orders	MIP: Chest pain	**Musculoskelatal ...**
Established by protocol	**Diagnosis ...**	Bone metastasis
Generated by physician	Dxs being considered **	Costochondritis
Access related care info	**Dxs not being considered ...**	Epidemic Myalgia
	Emergent **	Muscle strain/tear
	Non-emergent ...	Myofascial pain syndrome
	Esophageal **	Painful xiphoid syndrome
	Musculoskelatal **	Rib fracture
	Neurologic **	Slipping rib syndrome

The nurse does this by tapping on the last menu item on the first screen and then making a series of choices (next screen) that reveal a list of non-emergent, musculoskeletal disorders not yet considered (last screen). As shown in the following images …

< Davis, Michelle	< Davis, Michelle	< Davis, Michelle
Related care information	**Slipping rib syndrome**	**Slipping rib syndrome**

Related care information	Slipping rib syndrome	Slipping rib syndrome
Myofascial pain syndrome	**Findings**	**Finding related statement(s)**
Painful xiphoid syndrome	Pain: lower anterior costal margin (unilateral) intermittent sharp and severe somatic or visceral onset insidious	**Clicking sensation: reported or reproduced by hooking maneuver**
Rib fracture		
Slipping rib syndrome		The patient may report a painful clicking sensation, reproduced by hooking fingers under the affected costal margin and pulling anteriorly.
Sternalis syndrome	Tenderness and mobility: lower anterior ribs	
Thoracic spine segment dysfunction	Clicking sensation: reported or reproduced by hooking maneuver	
Thoracic spine compression fracture	pHx: trauma (remote)	
Tietze syndrome		

… after scrolling down to view all listed diagnoses, the nurse taps on "Slipping rib syndrome," which seems to be the most likely diagnosis given the pain location—the bottom of the rib cage, anteriorly. Doing so reveals related findings on the next screen. Because the specificity and/or sensitivity of findings for most *non-emergent* disorders have *not* been clearly established, the findings presented are *not* color-coded.

After viewing these findings, the nurse asks more questions and thereby learns that Michelle has experienced similar painful episodes in the same area, *not* immediately related to trauma, after injuring that area during a bicycle accident three years ago. The nurse then taps on the finding which is most specific for this disorder. Doing so reveals a related statement (last screen).

After performing this maneuver, which largely confirms the diagnosis, the nurse prompts further evaluation by the doctor, who then (1) documents the presence or absence of related checklist findings to explain and justify concluding that diagnosis as the main cause of Michelle's pain and (2) initiates recommended treatment.

Nurses might collaborate with physicians to improve diagnosis in other ways called for in the 2015 IOM report.

Permitting such doctor–nurse collaboration via shared use of the same evidence-based information can replace what is often a contentious, mutually demoralizing working environment with one that benefits doctors, nurses, and patients.

CHAPTER 5

Uneven Care Quality and Out-of-Control Costs—The Problem

THE INSTITUTE OF MEDICINE (IOM) was established in 1970 as an advisor to the US Congress by the National Academy of Sciences. It is now the National Academy of Medicine, one of three such academies in the United States—the National Academies of Sciences, Engineering, and Medicine. Like the others, the National Academy of Medicine is a private, nonprofit institution, which works outside the government to provide objective advice on matters related to medicine and health. It has more than 2,400 members elected by their peers in recognition of distinguished professional achievement. Membership criteria include

- distinguished achievement in a field within *or* related to medicine and health—related fields include natural, social, computational, and behavioral sciences as well as law, administration, and engineering;

- demonstrated and continued involvement with the issues of healthcare, prevention of disease, education, or research;

- skills and resources likely to contribute to achieving the Academy's mission; and

- willingness to be an active participant in the work of the Academy.

Three landmark IOM reports to Congress were published in 2000, 2001, and 2013:[57, 58, 59]

- *To Err Is Human: Building a Safer Health System*

- *Crossing the Quality Chasm: A New Health System for the 21st Century*

- *Best Care at Lower Cost: Path to Continuously Learning Healthcare in America*

The authors of the first report found that up to ninety-eight thousand US deaths each year likely resulted from preventable medical errors.[60] That report was transformational. It made headlines around the world. It also made care quality a political imperative, which paved the way for the publication of the second and third reports, which call for use of much better IT to address three interrelated problems:

- widespread physician burnout

- uneven care quality (adherence to evidence)

- out-of-control costs[61, 62]

More specifically, these reports call for fully integrated use of patient *and care* data within EHRs used to provide, document, and report care.

Two articles published twenty years after that first report describe progress toward improving care and reducing costs but also the need for a great deal more.[63, 64]

- "Two Decades Since *To Err Is Human*: An Assessment of Progress … " in *Health Affairs* (2018)

- "Two Decades Since *To Err Is Human*: Progress, but Still a 'Chasm'" in *JAMA* (2020)

The first article summarizes the need for more progress, stating: "In sum, the frequency of preventable harm remains high, and new scientific and policy approaches to address both prior and emerging risk areas are imperative…. This progress could lead us from a Bronze Age of rudimentary tool development to a Golden Era of vast improvement in patient safety."[65]

The second states: "In 2020, as a host of articles appeared to celebrate the anniversary of the report, the COVID-19 pandemic cruelly illustrated the ways in which the US health system has still fallen far short of the goal of providing safe, high-quality care."[66]

This chapter discusses the need to improve care quality and reduce costs per the recommendations in those IOM reports and recent publications. It also explains the relationship between those problems and physician burnout.

Chapter 6 explains how use of the IT called for in those publications can effectively address all three.

Need to Improve Care Quality, Defined as Adherence to Evidence

The second IOM report, *Crossing the Quality Chasm*, begins by stating: "The American health care delivery system is in need of fundamental change.... . Between the health care we have and the care we could have lies not just a gap, but a chasm." It points out that, while care for many individuals is excellent, "the health care delivery system has floundered in its ability to provide consistently high-quality care to all Americans" and further states, "If the health care system cannot consistently deliver today's science and technology, we may conclude that it is even less prepared to respond to the extraordinary scientific advances that will surely emerge during the first half of the 21st century." [67]

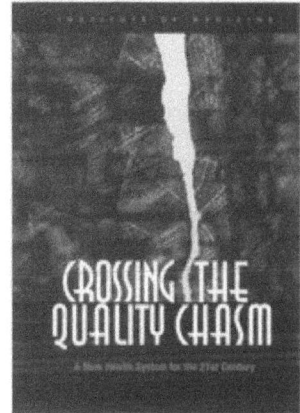

That report continues by stating, "The lag between the discovery of more efficacious forms of treatment and their incorporation into routine patient care is unnecessarily long ... Even then, adherence of clinical practice to the evidence is highly uneven ... the dissemination of guidelines alone has not been a very effective method of improving practice. Far more sophisticated clinical decision support systems will be needed ... "

It then defines a clinical decision support system as "software that integrates information on the characteristics of individual patients with a computerized knowledge base ... to aid clinicians and/or patients in making clinical decisions"[68] in other words, integrated use of patient *and care* data within EHRs.

EVIDENCE-BASED PRACTICE CLEARLY IMPROVES OUTCOMES

In a review article in *Worldviews on Evidence-Based Nursing*, published in February 2023, Linda Connor, PhD, RN, CPN, EBP-C and her colleagues reported the results of an exhaustive literature search and analysis that clearly demonstrates a positive correlation between EBP and improved outcomes. Of 8,537 articles or studies assessed, 636 that sufficiently examined that correlation were included for review. In the outcomes section of the article the authors state: "There were 1020 patient outcomes that were measured. Of the total patient outcomes measured, 908 (89.0%) improved, 104 (10.2%) showed no change, and eight (0.008%) worsened." Given the relatively few studies that met inclusion criteria, the authors called for more "coordinated and consistent use of established nomenclature and methods to evaluate EBP and patient outcomes." They concluded: "Leaders, clinicians, publishers, and educators all have a professional responsibility related to improving the current state of EBP."[69]

Crossing the Quality Chasm also notes, "More complex applications, such as computer-aided diagnosis, are in earlier stages of development, but the potential for these systems to contribute to evidence-based practice is great."[70]

Chapter 6 explains how use of computer-based, color-assisted, Bayesian-like analysis can do that by letting doctors fully process diagnostic data *and* fully integrate use of all patient and care data.

Need to Reduce Costs

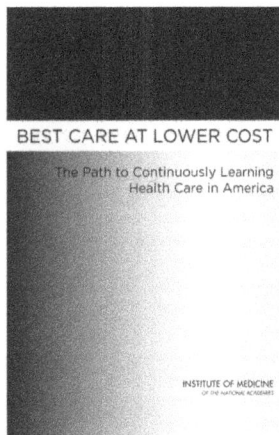

BEST CARE AT LOWER COST

The Path to Continuously Learning Health Care in America

INSTITUTE OF MEDICINE
OF THE NATIONAL ACADEMIES

The third IOM report, *Best Care at Lower Cost*, states, "For 31 of the past 40 years, health care costs [in the US] have increased at a greater rate than the economy as a whole … To put these cost increases into perspective, if the cost of other goods had risen as quickly as health care costs in the post–World War II period, a dozen eggs would now cost $55, a gallon of milk would cost $48, and a dozen oranges would cost $134."[71]

Current healthcare costs are bankrupting the US as a whole and millions of its individual citizens.

In a 2012 *Forbes* article titled "The U.S. Does Not Have a Debt Problem … It Has a Health Care Cost Problem," the author explains, "If health care costs were under control, i.e. growing no faster than the economy, we could manage our debt. However, health care spending is growing at about 1.5x the rate of growth of GDP and is already close to 20% of the economy." He then points out that if that trend continues,

- healthcare spending will eat up US GDP in our children's lifetimes;

- it will consume the federal government's budget even sooner, leaving no room for social security, defense, or any other government role; and

- therefore, "either taxes will rise to Swedish levels, or the U.S. will be a junk-quality sovereign credit" like the weakest economies during the European debt crisis.[72]

A 2024 report published by Paragon Health Institute sounded the alarm. Citing this report, the US Congressional Budget Office stated, "In 2024, federal spending on mandatory health programs—including Medicare, Medicaid, and Obamacare subsidies—is forecasted to reach $1.67 trillion. By 2033 federal spending on these health programs is projected to skyrocket to $3.103 trillion." They then pointed out, "By consuming a growing share of the federal budget, mandatory health care spending is the key driver of our nation's $34 trillion debt, driving America to the edge of insolvency. In fact, while other areas of federal spending are projected to decline in relation to GDP, spending on mandatory health programs is projected to rise … eating up more and more taxpayer dollars and wasting essential resources."[73]

State spending for education and other services is also being displaced. My state-supported medical education at the University of Utah cost me about eight thousand dollars. Per a November 2024 Education Data Initiative report, the current four-year cost for a Utah resident is about $203,000. The average four-year cost of public medical school education in the U.S. is about $215,000.[74]

Spending by US individuals is also a serious and growing problem. A 2024 Money article reported annual health insurance premiums in 2023 of $8,435 for single coverage and $23,968 for family coverage. While long-term projections are not available, the same article noted, each increased 7 percent in 2023 and was expected to increase another

6 percent in 2024.[75] Companies compensate for covering part of those premiums by increasing the cost of their goods or services, which contributes to overall inflation, or avoid premium costs by outsourcing labor to other countries. Also, a Kaiser Family Foundation study found that one in four adults—and six in ten uninsured adults—recently reported skipping or postponing medical care because of the cost.[76] Skipped or postponed care often increases future costs. Finally, according to a 2024 Governing report, about one hundred million Americans with or without insurance, who couldn't survive without care, were crippled by related debt.[77]

THE CAUSES OF OUT-OF-CONTROL COSTS

In a 2024 article published in *Annals of Bioethics & Clinical Applications*, the authors describe and discuss the main cause of these out-of-control costs. They note that, per Centers for Disease Control and Prevention estimates, more than 86 percent of US healthcare spending is related to chronic diseases, including heart disease, cancer, diabetes, stroke, and arthritis, and that most of these diseases are preventable. They further explain that while prevention is critical to the nation's economic well-being, it won't be easily achieved. Doing so would require eliminating or avoiding risk factors at a young age—most importantly, inactivity, poor diet, and smoking—and maintaining a healthy lifestyle thereafter.[78]

Most ED patients with chronic diseases seek care for exacerbations. Usually by that point the opportunity for prevention no longer exists. Like most doctors, ED physicians must therefore implement ways to manage acute diseases, including exacerbations of chronic diseases, more cost effectively.

In an article titled "The World's Costliest Health Care," David Cutler, Professor of Applied Economics, Harvard School of Public Health, discusses the three main causes of out-of-control costs in the US when caring for all patients: healthcare administrative costs, profiteering or price gouging, and overutilization of costly care.

He explains that administrative costs account for about one-third of healthcare spending, mainly because of the lack of standardization—every insurer requires the use of a unique barcode set and claim submission procedure.

Profiteering or price gouging is perpetuated in two ways. First, US providers charge much more for the same products or services than providers in other countries. Second, prestigious hospitals charge multiple times what other hospitals charge for the same care, including simple care such as routine x-rays.

Overutilization of costly care is largely caused by physician referral and/or patient desire for such care and under- or ineffective use of preventive care.[79]

A January 2024 article published by the Peter G. Peterson Foundation cites the same or similar reasons as those previously discussed:

- New, innovative technology can lead to better but more expensive procedures and products.

- The complexity of US healthcare can lead to administrative waste in insurance and provider payment systems.

- Consolidation of hospitals can lead to lack of competition or even a monopoly, granting providers the opportunity to increase prices.[80]

The IOM report *Best Care at Lower Cost* cites additional factors that contribute to high costs and/or waste, including

- the growing number and complexity of care options—especially those involving use of high technology, which strain or overwhelm human capacity to make cost-effective decisions;

- chronic diseases and comorbid conditions, which exacerbate the clinical, logistical, decision-making, and economic challenges faced by patients and clinicians; and

- the growing fragmentation of care, which compromises care provision or delivery.[81]

THE QUALITY PAYMENT PROGRAM

The US Quality Payment Program includes a shared savings program established in 2012 by the Centers for Medicare and Medicaid Services (CMS) to substantially reduce costs and improve quality by moving providers who agree to participate into accountable care organizations (ACOs). ACOs are groups of clinicians, hospitals, and other healthcare providers who come together voluntarily to give coordinated high-quality care to a designated group of patients. Those who document and report high-quality care and reduced care spending share Medicare program savings. The Pathways to Success program, implemented in 2019, offers a structured yet flexible "glide path" for ACOs as they take on increasing levels of performance-based financial risk.

Despite improved performance under Pathways to Success policies, participating ACOs have not achieved those objectives nearly as well as they could. Per the latest performance report, published by CMS in 2023, ACOs reduced net Medicare spending by $2.1 billion—only 0.21 percent of total Medicare spending (about $1 trillion).[82]

Furthermore, as shown in figure 4, per CMS published data, ACO participation in the program declined after those policies were implemented and has remained flat since then.[83]

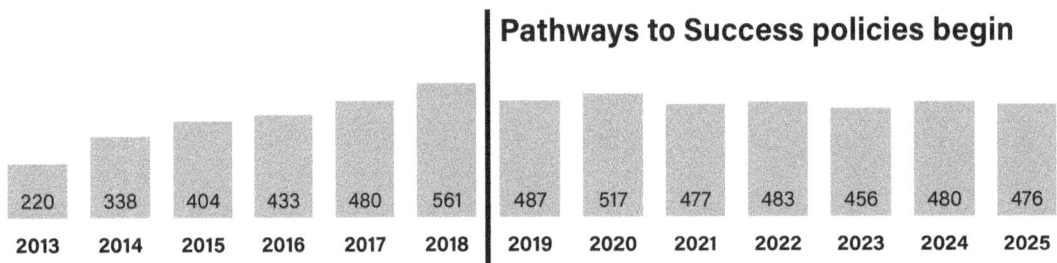

Pathways to Success policies begin

2013	2014	2015	2016	2017	2018	2019	2020	2021	2022	2023	2024	2025
220	338	404	433	480	561	487	517	477	483	456	480	476

Figure 4. Author created graph showing number of ACOs participating in the QPP shared savings program over time—based on a similar graph in an NAACOs article.[84]

One reason is that measuring and reporting quality measures, which may or may not improve care, is too expensive and time-consuming. A study reported in *Health Affairs* found physicians in four common specialties spent $15.4 billion in 2015 reporting quality measures.[85] A 2023 study found that reporting 162 quality measures at Johns Hopkins Hospital during calendar year 2018 required about 108,500 person-hours and cost a total of more than $5,640,000 for personnel costs and vendor fees.[86]

Most importantly, demand for provision and reporting of cost-effective care is accelerating physician burnout. Causes cited in chapter 1 are greatly compounded by such demand.

The IOM report *Crossing the Quality Chasm* explains the need for use of better IT to address burnout. It states, "Safety flaws are unacceptably common, but the effective remedy is not to browbeat the health care workforce by asking them to try harder ... Health care has safety and quality problems because it relies on outmoded systems of work. Poor design sets the workforce up to fail, regardless of how hard they try." It then calls for redesigned systems, including better IT, to support provision and reporting of cost-effective care.[87]

In a 2016 interview published in *Health Data Management*, Michael Hunt, MD, expressed frustration with demand for cost-effective care and the current state of IT. Dr. Hunt holds a master's degree in medical informatics and, at the time of the interview, was CEO and president of St. Vincent's Health Partners (SVHP) in Bridgeport, Connecticut. He spent more than ten years preparing to help SVHP become an ACO. During the interview, he stated, "Does anyone think those ACOs and physicians aren't trying their hardest … ? If you assume, like me, they are … then you have to think about the barriers to success."

He explained how complicated such care can be, even regarding the use of common procedures like mammograms, and added, "I think we've underestimated the complexity of … getting to where shared-savings programs want us to go. The practice of medicine is much more complex than it was a few years ago, and by not using IT to take some of that pressure off, we are disenfranchising physicians." He went on to explain why doctors don't need the best analytic platform ever built, but instead, IT that uses data to present "actionable information," which they can readily use to provide cost-effective care. He also stated that providing "the right care, at the right time, in the right environment will yield those cost savings … instead of directly focusing physicians on cutting costs."[88]

Chapter 6 describes how use of better IT can give physicians what Dr. Hunt asked for—immediate access to actionable information, produced via studies/analytics, while they're making decisions. Better IT can let them consistently provide (and report) the right care, at the right time, in the right environment, *and at the best price*, to improve quality and reduce costs at every care point.

CHAPTER 6

Uneven Care Quality and Out-of-Control Costs—The Solution

THE HIPUS® SYSTEM is well designed to improve care quality and reduce costs:

- Physicians largely determine care quality and generate the bulk of spending by their decisions.

- Besides prevention, early, accurate, and precise diagnosis is the single best way to reduce costs without rationing care.

- Color-assisted, Bayesian-like analysis will let doctors fully process diagnostic data and thereby improve diagnosis.

- Doctors make almost all decisions to arrive at (rule in or out) or respond to (treat or prevent) a diagnosis.

- Linking all other care data (costs of and indications for tests, referrals, treatments, and hospitalizations) and/or AI or ML products to diagnoses (disorders) or diagnostic assistance (findings) is the best way to make that data immediately available while doctors and patients are making decisions.

- Care and patient data stored within an RDB will permit fully integrated use.

- Highly modular care and patient data processed via well-designed applications can be used to do pretty much anything that might be imagined. Astonishing internet-based search engines, maps, travel guides, and other products are examples of that.

The importance of color-coded diagnostic data is hard to overstate. With it, doctors can fully process diagnostic data and fully integrate use of all patient and care data. Without it, they can't do either. In a letter to then Pennsylvania Governor Ed Rendell (chapter 7), a software designer referred to use of such data as "an invention which may well be a missing cog in the machine of medicine in not only this state, but the world."

Improving Care Quality

Giving physicians immediate access to evidence-based data while they're making decisions and letting them use it with relative ease and speed can greatly improve care quality.

Letting physicians use that same data to easily or automatically document and report care quality can dramatically reduce the time needed to do so.

The same data used to provide and report care can facilitate better studies or analysis needed to further improve care.

Reducing Care Costs

Highly modular patient and care data processed via well-designed applications can effectively address the main causes of excess care spending, particularly administrative costs, profiteering or price gouging, and overutilization of costly care. While additional measures will be needed—for example, mandating use of standardized barcodes and procedures when submitting insurance claims—use of better IT is essential to addressing those causes.

Administrative costs: Better IT that lets physicians readily document and report cost-effective care in ways easily understood and accepted by payers can also be used to automatically submit claims via standardized use of barcodes and procedures.

Profiteering or price gouging: Better IT that lets physicians and patients easily shop for cost-effective care *while making decisions* can drive costs down via the same market forces that determine pricing in other industries. It can also do so by detailing and exposing exorbitant pricing and thereby propel reform to address that problem.

Overutilization of costly care: When combined with the right incentives, letting patients readily shop for cost-effective care while making decisions can also prevent overuse of needless or needlessly expensive care. Also, because disease prevention is the best way to lower utilization, widespread use of better IT to improve prevention can dramatically reduce spending.

How HIPUS® System Use Can Reduce Care Costs—Two Examples

The following examples describe, in part, coordinated evaluation and management of acute otitis media (middle ear infection) in Eric Coleman, a five-year-old, by an emergency physician and a primary care physician. Admittedly, providing the care described is a relatively simple undertaking. But again, use of highly modular patient and care data and well-designed applications can permit cost-effective care of much more complicated conditions involving new technology, chronic diseases, and comorbidity and let a variety of different specialists in different settings better coordinate care.

Screen 1

< Coleman, Eric

Final diagnosis:

Acute otitis media: ped

Select:

Document presence or absence of associated disorders.

Provide initial or further treatment.

OTHER *

Screen 2

< Coleman, Eric

Ear pain • 5 YR M • 1:45 AM ♀ 4   ○

i   Dx   **Tx**

Generate

Orders **

Prescriptions

Discharge Instructions

Document

Tx Procedures

Patient Response

Disposition

Randomly Access Tx Info

Screen 3

< Coleman, Eric

Prescriptions

Options presented are for isolated AOM

Select:

Analgesics

Antibiotics

OTHER *

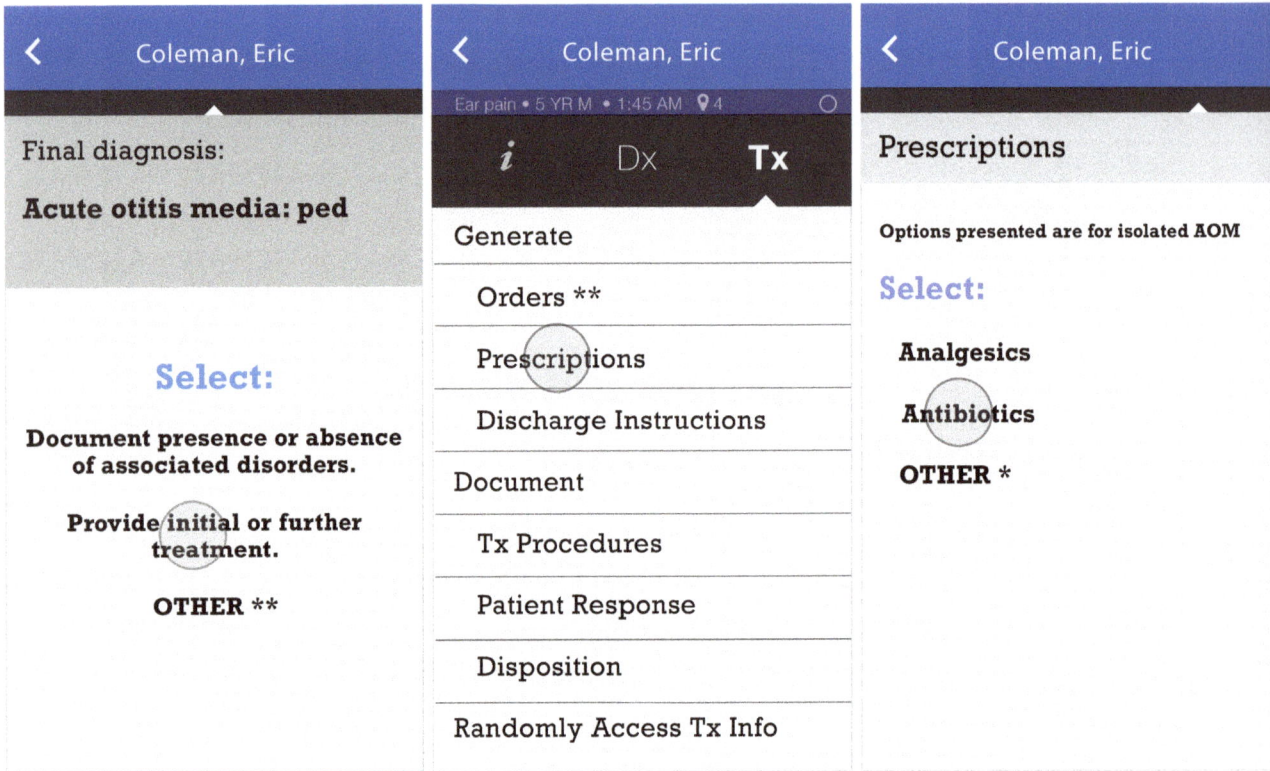

After using the HIPUS® system to conclude the diagnosis shown at the top of the first screen—acute otitis media (middle ear infection)—the emergency physician selects the second option presented and then uses the treatment (Tx) menu (next screen) to initiate or resume treatment by choosing to generate a prescription. By tapping on "Antibiotics" (third screen) and then indicating the treatment setting—initial treatment of an acute episode (not shown here) …

< Coleman, Eric	< Coleman, Eric	< Coleman, Eric

Prescriptions: antibiotic

Select drug: Cost

Amoxicillin $11-41

Amoxicillin-Clavulanate $26-48

Cephalosporins (5) **

Clindamycin $12-48

OTHER via... ⌨ 🎤

Generic Brand

Prescriptions: antibiotic

Amoxicillin $11-41 MED √ CLEAR

Recommended regimen for pt weight of 42 lbs:16-1800 mg/day div q12h x 7 days

Select preparation:

400 mg / 5 ml sus 5oz

400 mg tab chew #30

500 mg capsule #24

500 mg tablet #24

875 mg tablet #14

Prescriptions: antibiotic

Amoxicillin $13-35 SHOP

Recommended regimen for pt weight of 42 lbs:16-1800 mg/day div q12h x 7 days

Select preparation:

400 mg / 5 ml susp 5oz

400 mg tab chew #30

500 mg capsule #24

500 mg tablet #24

875 mg tablet

Generate Rx

… the physician accesses a list of antibiotic choices recommended by the American Academy of Pediatrics and the cost range for generic drugs. Generic drugs are always presented initially—brand-name options are presented only if the physician chooses to view them. The system thereby prompts routine use of equally effective and much less expensive generic drugs. The physician selects amoxicillin, the first-line recommendation. As shown at the top of the second screen, the system then

- presents again the name and cost range of the selected drug;

- checks for possible adverse drug reactions, given the presence of co-occurring disorders and/or other drugs being used by the patient, and presents the results of that check (brown font, right upper corner); and

- presents a recommended drug regimen, given the patient's weight and need for any adjustments identified by the drug check.

As shown on the last two screens, it then presents a list of available drug preparations and the needed volume or number of each given that recommended regimen. When Eric's mother selects chewable tabs, the physician taps on it. The system then presents the cost range for that preparation and invites Mrs. Coleman to shop for the best price at a pharmacy she wants to use. Because she pays for meds out of pocket, she chooses to do that. When the physician taps on "SHOP," …

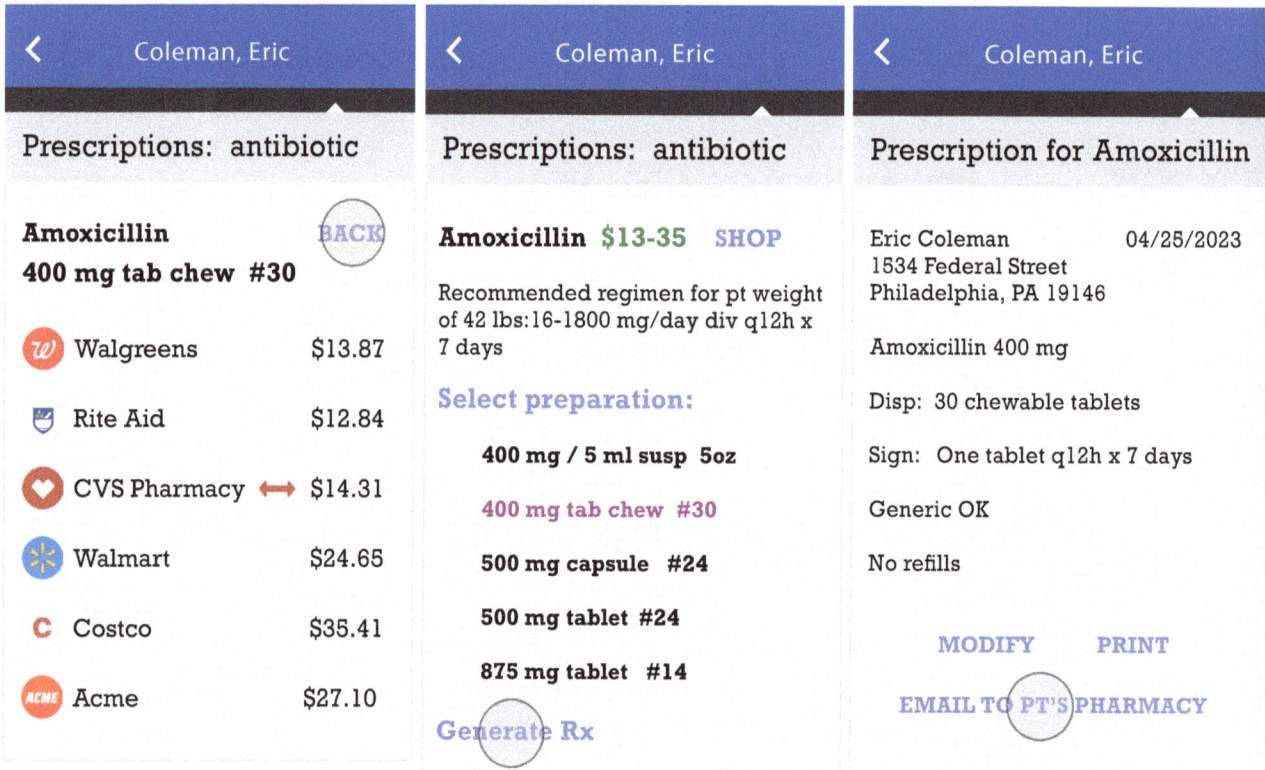

‹ Coleman, Eric

Prescriptions: antibiotic

Amoxicillin   BACK
400 mg tab chew #30

W Walgreens $13.87

R Rite Aid $12.84

♥ CVS Pharmacy ⟷ $14.31

✴ Walmart $24.65

C Costco $35.41

ACME Acme $27.10

‹ Coleman, Eric

Prescriptions: antibiotic

Amoxicillin $13-35   SHOP

Recommended regimen for pt weight of 42 lbs:16-1800 mg/day div q12h x 7 days

Select preparation:

  400 mg / 5 ml susp 5oz

  400 mg tab chew #30

  500 mg capsule #24

  500 mg tablet #24

  875 mg tablet #14

Generate Rx

‹ Coleman, Eric

Prescription for Amoxicillin

Eric Coleman   04/25/2023
1534 Federal Street
Philadelphia, PA 19146

Amoxicillin 400 mg

Disp: 30 chewable tablets

Sign: One tablet q12h x 7 days

Generic OK

No refills

       MODIFY   PRINT

   EMAIL TO PT'S PHARMACY

… the system again presents the drug name, preparation, and number of needed tablets. It also presents the price of those tablets at each of six local pharmacies. Because $14.31 is close to the lowest price and Mrs. Coleman routinely obtains meds at one of CVS's stores, she tells the doctor she wants to use the preparation sold by that pharmacy. As shown on the next two screens, the physician then returns to the previous menu and prompts the system to generate a prescription, which they email to that store.

About a month later, Eric's mother takes him to see his primary doctor for a routine visit. The following describes use of a desktop computer and HIPUS® applications.

The same EHR founder and president who provided time and cost estimates for incorporating *mobile* physician assistance into a preexisting EDIS (chapter 2) provided estimates for incorporating *desktop* physician assistance into a preexisting primary care EHR—also about six months and $500,000.

One reason cited for ACO failure to reduce spending as much as was hoped for is that most hospitals and physicians have not been able to tightly coordinate care.[89] The following shows how that might be addressed by letting any physician within an ACO contribute to and/or access the total medical record of all patients within that ACO.

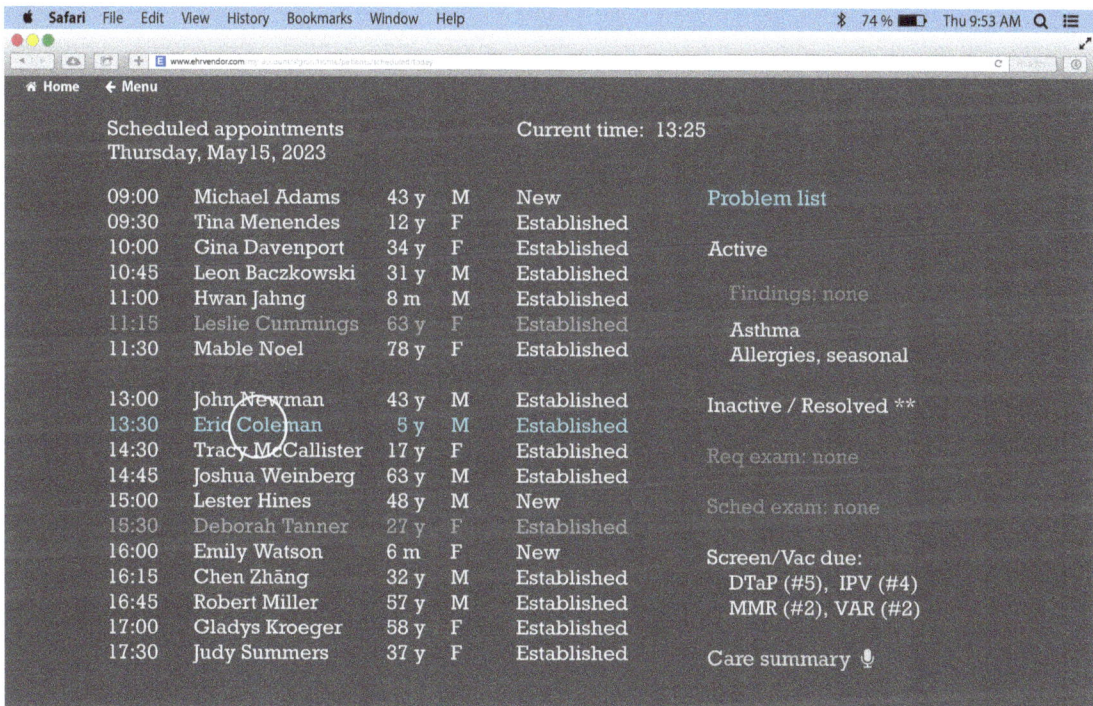

Shortly before seeing Eric and his mother, the physician quickly reviews the problem list, including vaccinations now needed. When they arrive, she clicks on Eric's name.

As the following image shows …

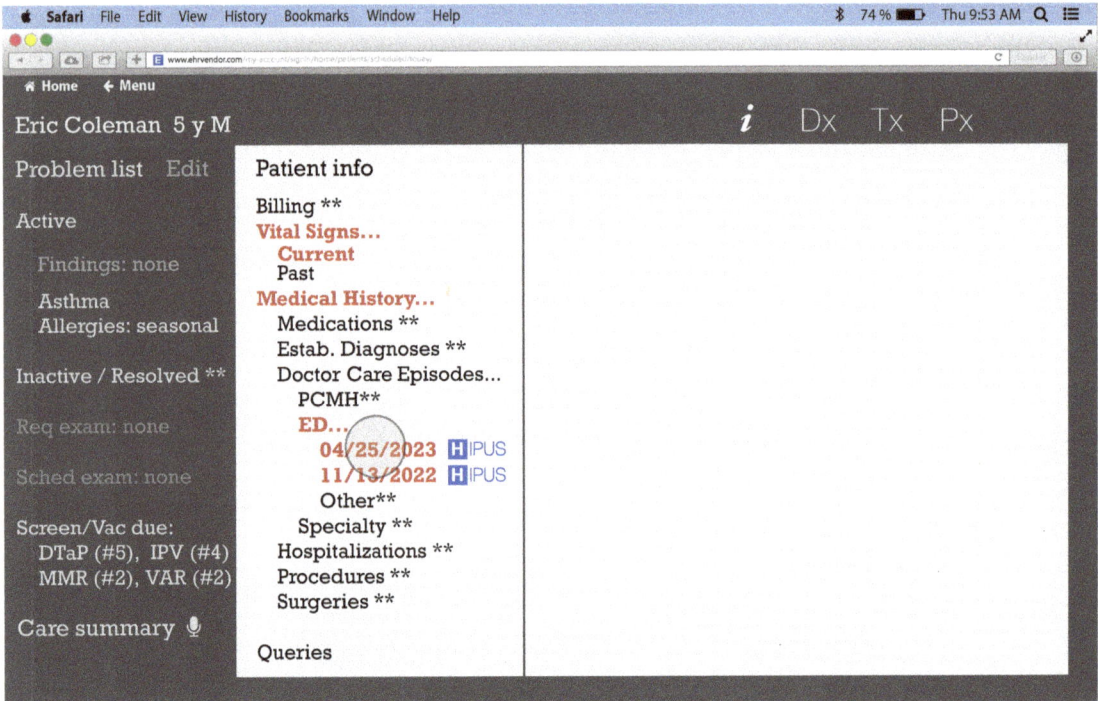

… the physician can then use the same set of menus shown in chapter 2 (used by ED physicians) as well as a Prevention (Px) menu. After conversing with Eric and his mother about his ED care for ear infections, the physician uses the patient info (i) menu to access Eric's medical record. Info added since his last visit is highlighted, including his vital signs obtained by the nurse and records of those ED care episodes produced via the HIPUS® system. After viewing Eric's vital signs, she selects the first record, which describes that care episode.

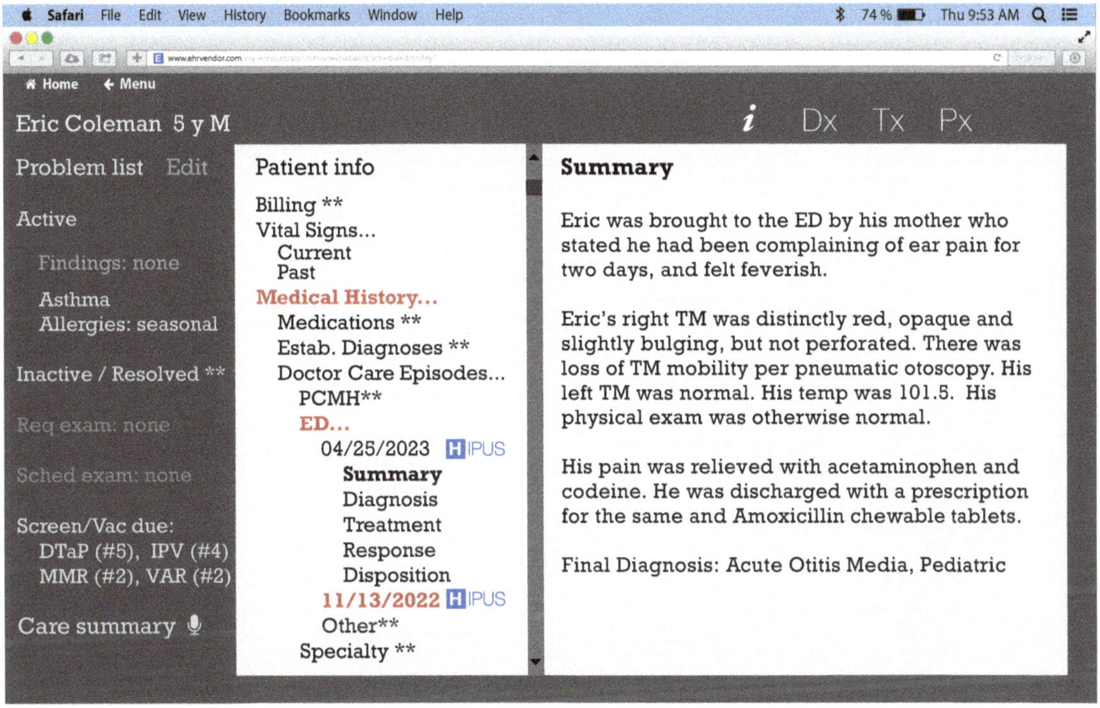

This record was produced using the same standardized methods described in chapter 2. After reading the ED physician's dictated care summary, the physician views diagnosis-related info (not shown here). She finds the ED physician's diagnosis of acute otitis media to be credible, given the well-documented use of a complete set of relevant findings and methods for determining the presence or absence of each, as recommended by the American Academy of Pediatrics. The physician then views the record of the previous ED care episode and learns that Eric has had two well-documented ear infections within six months. Eric's mother reports that he was also treated by a doctor for an ear infection while visiting his grandmother during the holidays. The physician therefore concludes that Eric, by definition, has *recurrent* acute otitis media (three infections within six months).

As shown on the next screen …

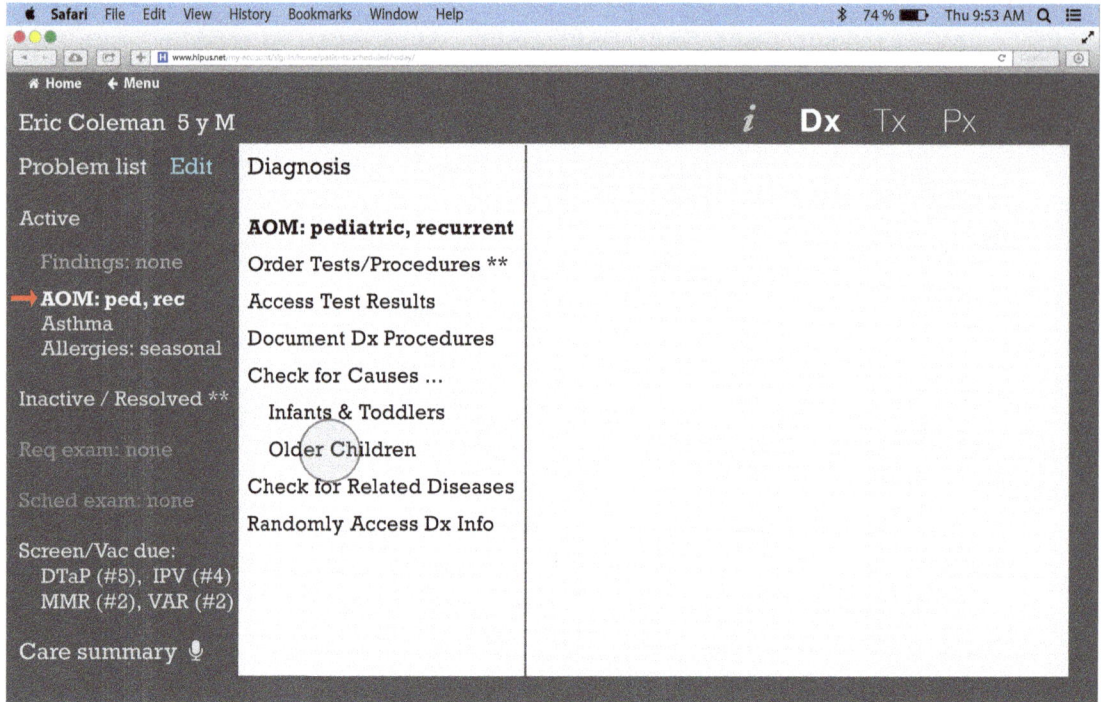

… the physician updates Eric's problem list to include that diagnosis (→), and then, using the diagnosis (Dx) menu, selects "Check for Causes" and then "Older Children."

As shown in the next image …

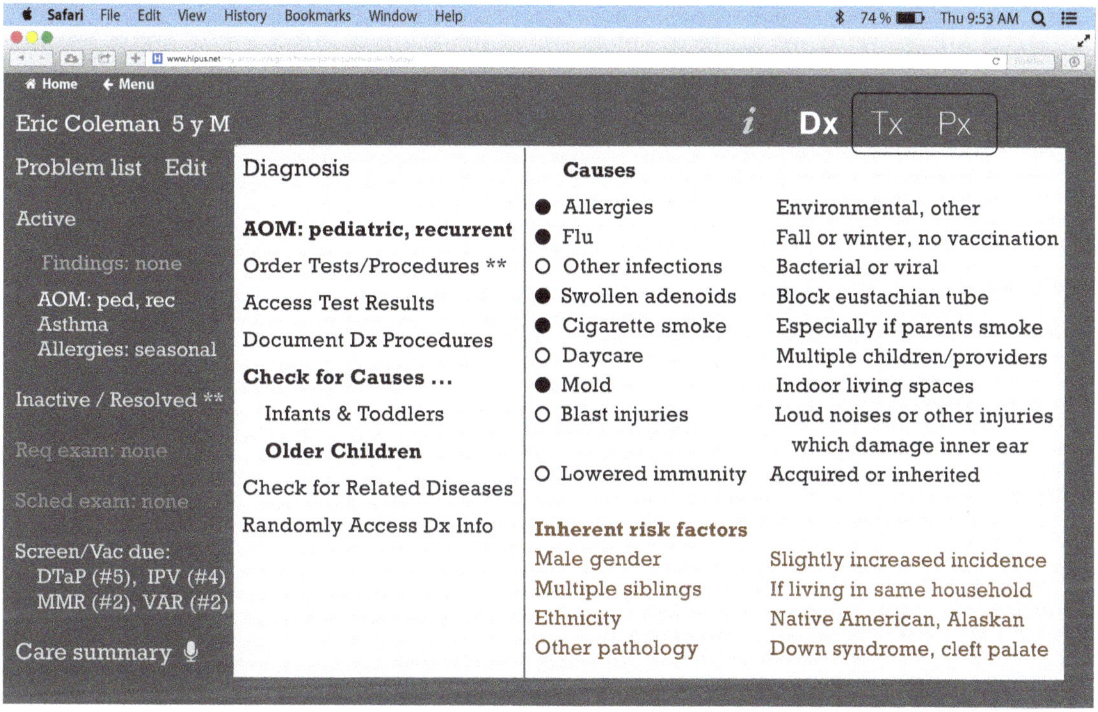

... doing so reveals a list of causes or risk factors. Most shown here are more important with infants or toddlers but also warrant consideration with older children. The physician works through them by discussing each possible cause with Eric's mother:

- Eric's seasonal allergies (see problem list) are usually a problem in late spring and early summer. His mother, however, reports what seem like allergic symptoms starting last fall, which prompts the physician to review info about winter allergies in the HIPUS® knowledge base, thereby recalling that they're usually due to mold spores,* dust mites, and/or pet dander. The family has no other members with similar symptoms and no pets, which makes dust mites and pet dander unlikely causes. Eric's mother suspects mold may be the culprit. Eric's bedroom is in the basement, and she discovered what appears to be mold in his room.

- After discussing the second cause, Eric's mother agrees to a flu vaccination.

---

* Mold spores are irritants as well as allergens and are therefore presented as a separate cause.

- His mother doesn't recall Eric having any signs or symptoms of upper respiratory tract infections along with his ear infections, and ED records don't report any.

- The physician examines Eric's adenoids using a special mirror and finds that they are mildly swollen.

- His mother commits to smoking less, and not at all in Eric's living spaces.

No other causes are identified. The causes or risk factors at the bottom of the screen can't be eliminated, but the only one present is Eric's gender, which is insignificant.

The physician and Eric's mother agree to address three potential causes or contributing factors—mold spores, flu, and cigarette smoke—to see if doing so prevents more ear infections and reduces adenoid swelling. If doing so doesn't prevent more infections, and adenoid swelling is the same or worse, Eric will be referred to an ear, nose, and throat specialist for possible adenoid removal.

The physician then uses the treatment (Tx) and prevention (Px) menus to document steps taken to address all of the previously listed potential causes, including

- renewing prescriptions for asthma and spring allergies, which Eric can also use during other seasons to treat similar symptoms caused by mold spores;

- obtaining a blood sample, sending it to a lab for mold sensitivity testing, and notifying Eric's mother about the results;

- providing instructions about ways to remove household mold, accessed via a HIPUS®- recommended website;

- obtaining parental consent for and scheduling a flu vaccination in September;

- documenting the mother's expressed commitment to reducing and modifying cigarette use; and

- scheduling a follow-up appointment in September.

Over time, that preventive care may preclude the need for much more expensive care, including more ED visits for ear infections, insertion of ear tubes, adenoid removal, and management of serious complications including hearing impairment and infection-related damage to adjacent tissue and/or organs.

The care described in this chapter illustrates the following points:

The money Mrs. Coleman saved might not seem like much to most people, but widespread use of similar applications to shop for much more expensive products and services *while doctors and patients are making decisions* can reduce overall healthcare spending tremendously. In a 2024 article, the authors describe growing efforts by healthcare regulators to increase pricing transparency, which can unleash market forces to increase competition, decrease healthcare expenditures, and provide widespread access to affordable, high-quality care.[90] A FAIR Health website at fairhealthconsumer.org provides ready access to zip code–dependent prices for a wide variety of goods and services. It does so using a database containing more than **forty-six billion private healthcare claim records** and **forty-five billion Medicare claim records** for **ten thousand services** in all areas of the United States dating back to **2002**.[91]

Care reports that can be readily understood and accepted by not only healthcare providers but also payers can expedite reimbursement. Submitting such reports along with invoices or claims using standardized procedures and barcodes can reduce administrative costs. Over time, demonstrated physician ability to readily explain and justify care can reduce payer-required preauthorizations.

Widespread use of better technology to help doctors coordinate preventive care and render it more effective can greatly reduce widespread spending for costly, avoidable care.

The primary care physician had ready access to not only Eric's ED care records but also the HIPUS® knowledge base and HIPUS® recommended web-based info, which the physician otherwise might not have recalled and/or been able to access while caring for Eric and fifteen other pediatric and/or adult patients that day.

Chapters 7 and 8 explain why doctor fear of change is the main barrier to implementing needed IT, and what you, as a doctor *or nonphysician*, can do to propel needed change.

CHAPTER 7

Doctor Fear of Needed Change

IN 2000, I PRESENTED the HIPUS® system to a US EM professional organization board member who later became its president. His first response was "Doctors are scared to death of change." I've since learned that he wasn't exaggerating. I have also found, with few exceptions, that doctors can't or won't talk about it.

What I Found to Be the Cause

Again, US physicians spend a huge amount of time, money, and effort to acquire a medical education and become board-certified and therefore rightly expect that to be enough.

They become board-certified partly by memorizing a huge amount of information to pass a test. Certification, which implies an ability to process that info appropriately whenever needed, has been used to justify physician status and income for generations. Needed change (discussed in chapters 1 and 2), which implies otherwise, devalues certification, in the minds of most doctors, intolerably.

US physicians have been powerfully conditioned in that and other ways* to believe that they are somehow different from other professionals and therefore needn't use IT the way others use it to survive. They *have* started using apps to calculate risk for heart disease, fracture (given osteoporosis), and other potential problems and to perform certain tasks such as prescribing drugs. But resistance to use of IT to improve diagnosis—the most important task, which more than any other defines the medical profession and can improve IT use in every other way—remains entrenched.

That belief is a hugely important part of how most US physicians see themselves, but it doesn't withstand examination. Most doctors therefore can't or won't talk about it.

While an attempt to describe how problematic fear of change is, this chapter is *not* an attempt to attach blame. I found such fear to be nearly universal and the product of many years of conditioning. I also understand how powerful conditioning can be. Realizing that my being gay would never change nearly killed me. I survived by talking about it and taking deliberate steps to come to terms with it. What physicians are now experiencing seems, in some ways, to be a similar crisis. I hope this book will encourage doctors to do the same.

This chapter describes the radically different responses to the HIPUS® project by health-care pioneers and nonphysicians compared to doctors and presents examples of how doctor response helped produce and now sustains physician burnout. It concludes by explaining why doctors needn't fear such change.

Radically Different Responses to the HIPUS® Project

The following well-documented responses fairly represent numerous similar responses.

---

*   Those ways include: TV doctors shows from the 1950s to the present day that portray doctors as being different from other professionals; use of white coats that convey the same message; and universal use of "Doctor" or "Dr." when referring to physicians compared to nonuse or inconsistent use of that and other titles when referring to PhDs and other professionals.

US HEALTHCARE PIONEER RESPONSE

The following pioneers who lead the way into other uncharted waters expressed great interest in the HIPUS® project after viewing related material.

- **Homer Warner, MD, PhD.** Dr. Warner served as (1) the first president of the American College of Medical Informatics, (2) editor of the journal *Computers and Biomedical Research*, and (3) a senior member of the IOM. He was the first to recommend patent protection for the color-coded interface. He also asked me to work with him to develop computer-based diagnostic assistance at the University of Utah (my alma mater). For several reasons, I chose not to do so and instead moved from Salt Lake City to Philadelphia to continue working on the HIPUS® project. He responded by opening doors for me at several medical centers from New York City to Washington, DC.

- **Paul Clayton, PhD.** Dr. Clayton was a professor and director at the Center for Medical Informatics at Columbia-Presbyterian Medical Center. He invited me to present my ideas to "about twenty people interested in building hospital information systems with automated decision-making capabilities." He did so at the behest of Dr. Henrik Bendixen, dean of Columbia University College of Physicians and Surgeons, who likely discussed my ideas with Dr. Warner. I declined for reasons related to my patent application.

- **Carol Rivers, MD.** Dr. Rivers was one of the first EM residents in the US. She went on to edit and publish preparatory textbooks for EM board exams. Dr. Rivers strongly endorsed use of the color-coded interface and the HIPUS® system generally (see chapter 2). She also endorsed a knowledge base I constructed for acute coronary syndrome (heart attack and UA) variations.

- **Eta Berner, EdD.** Dr. Berner led a team of thirteen MD/PhDs who evaluated the performance of four computer-based systems built by the US medical informatics community to replace doctors as expert diagnosticians or let them be active, information-seeking participants in the diagnostic process (see chapter 3). Her study was published as a special article in *The New England Journal of Medicine*. She sent me a three-page, single-spaced email response to HIPUS® material, expressing great interest in the color-coded interface.

- **Alan Somers, MPH, MBA, JD.** Mr. Somers earned a master's degree in health management and policy at the University of Michigan, then ranked the number one program of its kind by *U.S. News & World Report*. He then developed all policies, systems, procedures, and contracts needed by the health maintenance organization (HMO) HealthPlus of Michigan to manage its quality and costs. As VP for managed care, he selected strategic allies from twenty-six HMOs and preferred provider organizations for the US's fifth largest municipal hospital chain. Alan strongly endorsed and assisted my efforts to implement the HIPUS® system.

NONPHYSICIAN OR LAY RESPONSE

With few exceptions, presènting the HIPUS® system to nonphysicians elicited animated conversations. They asked good questions, understood the need for it, and very much wanted doctors to use it.

The following responses are not intended as a substitute for a well-designed and carefully interpreted survey covering lay response to actual use of the HIPUS® system. They do, however, provide examples of patient frustration with current care and desire for better approaches.

PENNSYLVANIA GOVERNOR ED RENDELL'S RESPONSE

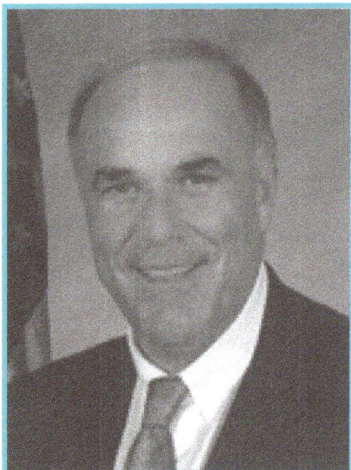

In September 2002, during Governor Rendell's first gubernatorial campaign, at one of six fundraisers he attended that evening, I showed him the back of my business card, which stated:

- Product: Patented, palmtop, color-coded diagnostic assistance

- Market: HMOs

- Service: Giving doctors *immediate* access to diagnostic and other cost saving information *while they're making decisions*

and said to him, "I believe this can help you and Pennsylvania."

I then sent him a follow-up letter. He responded by inviting me to meet with his issues and policy director. When I entered her office, she offered me twenty minutes. We conversed for more than an hour. Afterward, I was invited to all the inaugural events, including a fairly exclusive Governor's open house. When I sent Rendell a note thanking him for that, he responded: "Thanks for your kind note and all your help. I don't intend to let you down." About a month later, for reasons not explained, he withdrew support for the HIPUS® project. I suspect he encountered the same entrenched resistance to change I encountered over twenty years.

OTHER NONPHYSICIAN RESPONSES

Rendell's expressed interest, however, prompted me to recruit other nonphysicians to help me produce material that might be used to elicit his administration's financial, political, and/ or administrative support for the project. Those nonphysicians helped me produce a related website, CD-ROM slideshow, and demo prototype in three months. Their interest in and desire for physician use of the HIPUS® system was so intense that I had to work very hard to keep up with them. They and others who viewed that material sent Rendell letters urging his continued support. I got the idea for those letters from Lisa, an IRS agent who audited my tax returns, claiming large deductions for HIPUS®-related business expenses. After doing so, she declared her intention to send Rendell such a letter *without being asked*. The others barely had to be asked.

They were as different as the letters they wrote.

Rob was (or still is) a software developer.

Judith was a retail brand manager for Aramark Campus Services.

Marlene was seventy-eight and had recently launched a modeling career.

Roy was a sound designer, recording engineer, and audio producer/director.

Joe was a photographer.

Jonathan was a website designer with expertise in PDAs.

Lisa was an IRS agent.

Joanna was a website designer with a law degree.

But they all understood the need for such assistance and wanted their doctors to use it.

- Rob wrote: "Though somewhat jaded by thirty-six years of dealing with cutting-edge technology, Pennsylvania's own Dr. Mark Sorensen has impressed me by bringing forth an invention which may well be a missing cog in the machine of medicine in not only this state, but the world. Dr. Sorensen has invented a way to enable medical personnel to make better decisions and make them faster and more accurately than ever before. I believe the state in which Dr. Sorensen happens to reside when his invention takes hold will be viewed as a technology hub much in the way of Silicon Valley."

- Judith wrote: "I am a [healthcare] consumer who has undergone countless unnecessary medical tests, which have been very costly to both my insurance company and myself. Besides the cost, the stress of going through these tests and the time spent waiting in hospitals has also affected my life. I'm curious about why we're not already utilizing this exciting tool."

- Marlene wrote: "For the past eight months my family has been in constant turmoil. My husband of forty-eight years underwent the surgical removal of his large toe. Prior to this drastic procedure it was REFERRAL after REFERRAL! Then came DIAGNOSIS after DIAGNOSIS! Finally, PRESCRIPTION after PRESCRIPTION! This is STILL ongoing as the healing is in process. I am a vintage model/actor dedicated to my beloved spouse. With HIPUS®, integration of all the above would give me peace of mind and the time to pursue my career. I strongly recommend that you take a hard look at HIPUS® and request implementation in the state of Pennsylvania and nationwide."

- Roy wrote: "For the past two years, I've been struggling with a condition which involves a cardiologist, an endocrinologist, an electrophysiologist, and my primary health care provider. It's a long story of confusion and money not well spent. After studying the HIPUS® website AND producing voice over for *Concluding and Responding to a Diagnosis*, I now realize an accurate diagnosis could have been concluded expeditiously. All physicians could have been using the same information (supported by studies) and would have identified the least costly method of treatment. HIPUS® is important to the future of healthcare because it creates a win-win situation for everyone."

- Joe wrote: "The solutions offered at www.hipus.net seem very promising. I have experienced bloated costs, ridiculous paperwork, and other healthcare inefficiencies and distortions, as well as loss of the 'human touch' in our healthcare system. The ideas proposed seem to give the physician cost-saving information exactly when needed. It could free an inefficient system to attend more to the human side of healthcare. Costs could be reduced. Accuracy of treatment could be increased."

- Jonathan wrote: "As a consumer of healthcare, and as an owner of a small technology business, HIPUS® will have a profound effect on me and my family. HIPUS® is an idea whose time has come. The opportunities for improving the quality and cost of healthcare along with the potential for developing businesses cannot be ignored."

- Lisa wrote: "Dr. Sorensen has spent many years developing and perfecting HIPUS® to aid physicians and alleviate the financial and physical cost of misdiagnosis. I personally do not know anyone who would not feel safer in the hands of physicians if their skills were enhanced with a device such as HIPUS®."

- Joanna wrote: "Having trained and practiced in more than one information-intensive profession, I can see that the 'practice' of medicine needs more skillful means to keep relevant information available, yet not overwhelming, at the immediate point of service. The patented approach shown at www.hipus.net seems to offer a unique and human-friendly solution."

Numerous other nonphysician responses were equally positive. The following are examples.

- The dean of West Chester University's business school (in Pennsylvania) learned about the HIPUS® project through his association with Alan Somers. After viewing related material, he invited me to spend time talking about it. During our one-hour meeting he talked, nonstop, about the project as a business venture. I could barely get a word in edgewise. I had to end the meeting by walking out of his office. While I did so, he was still talking about it.

- After producing a HIPUS® promotional video with Speed Graphics in New York City, because I didn't have a VCR, I viewed the finished product using one in the lobby of a DoubleTree hotel in downtown Philadelphia. While doing so, I didn't notice that a security guard was also viewing it. After he viewed it for not more than ten minutes he said to me: "Did you do this? Doctors are just guessing. If they use this, they won't be guessing. If I had a hundred thousand dollars, I'd invest in this thing right now."

- At a Silicon Valley venture capital summit in New York City, I presented the HIPUS® project to about twenty venture capitalists (VCs). Because I had to present the project to each in less than five minutes, I did so the same way I had presented it to Ed Rendell—using the back of the same business card. Nine out of ten VCs with medical products in their portfolios expressed interest. Three expressed serious interest, including one whose business partner who delivered the keynote address at that conference and whose firm managed a $7 billion international portfolio. After viewing the back of my card, he asked for "hard copy," which was highly unusual—everyone else wanted emails. When the crowd around him dispersed, the document I gave him was the only thing in his hand. The most candid VC response, however, explains why nothing resulted from those encounters. This individual said to me, "No one has penetrated healthcare."

After collaborating with a series of nonphysicians, I and several of those collaborators are now prepared to implement the HIPUS® system. I was told by a National Institute of Health (NIH) Small Business Innovation Research (SBIR) grant program officer that the project is an eligible candidate for up to $3 million in US federal grant money as a potentially effective way to address physician burnout and related problems. Before submitting a formal proposal requesting grant money, I need to persuade an EM professional organization to participate in the project.

PHYSICIAN RESPONSES

Presenting the system to US board-certified physicians in various ways—face-to-face conversations, emails with attachments, websites, etc.—elicited little or no response.

Again, being the product of powerful long-term conditioning, their nonresponse was nearly universal.

Those physicians included

- colleagues I interacted with while doing locum tenens work in numerous EDs;

- physicians serving as HMO, ACO, and hospital executives, med school deans, residency directors, CME providers, EHR vendor executives, and innovation center staff; and

- numerous physicians attending an annual conference of an EM professional organization.

Colleague response was generally hostile and not explained. The most striking responses, elicited from a few who were somewhat compelled to explain, were variations of "I can't remember the meanings of the colors." To use the system, one need remember the meanings of only four colors. Physicians memorize thousands of facts to pass board exams.

A handful of the physician leaders responded *briefly*—the rest, not at all.

While attending the EM professional organization conference, I handed out about 120 business cards inviting doctors to view a five-minute slideshow on their phones explaining need for color-assisted, Bayesian-like analysis and provide a response. I received no responses per phone, and only one face-to-face response—a brief response from that organization's president who viewed the slide show.

DOCTOR FEAR OF CHANGE HELPED PRODUCE AND NOW SUSTAINS PHYSICIAN BURNOUT

While preparing to implement the HIPUS® system, I found that doctor fear of needed change is the only obstacle to doing so.

Such Fear Helped Produce and Now Sustains EHR Dysfunction

After reading the IOM report *Crossing the Quality Chasm*, which calls for fully integrated use of patient and care data within EHRs,[92] and seeing that two HMO executives were on the committee who produced it, Alan Somers (the previously named healthcare pioneer) and I sent those executives material explaining how that objective might be achieved. We did so three times, which finally elicited a phone conversation with one mid-level HMO representative. After briefly summarizing the material, I said, "I'm just asking you to keep an open mind." He responded, "Of course, but I can't be responsible for how doctors might respond to a new idea." When he said that his voice changed, the way voices do when people are afraid, and with that, the conversation ended. Again, EHR vendors then gave doctors what they wanted—as much as possible, *no change* to the way they provide, document, and report care by processing diagnostic info from memory only. For reasons cited in chapter 1, not long after physicians began using those EHRs, they came to hate what they had asked for.

A physician, while on the AMA board of directors, spent two or three years demanding useable EHRs, but when I tried to discuss how they might be rendered more useable per those IOM report recommendations, he couldn't or wouldn't discuss it.

Again, the 21st Century Cures Act (discussed in chapter 1) was enacted by the US Congress, partly to help make EHRs more useable. It can only achieve that objective, however, if providers—hospitals or physicians—request use of new technology. Physicians have ample reasons to use such technology but fear the needed change too much to do so.

Such Fear Nixed a Solid Proposal to Build the HIPUS® System

While attending that EM professional organization conference, I attended a workforce-related session during which members discussed what they clearly found to be serious causes of burnout, including those described in chapter 1.

Immediately after that session, during my brief conversation with that organization's president, he reported viewing the five-minute slideshow and stated, "This needs to be done. We need to do this."

After a longer conversation with another board member who then viewed the slideshow, I was invited to submit a formal proposal to that organization's entire board of directors, asking them to consider collaborating with HIPUS, LLC to implement and test the study product described in the slideshow. That proposal presented a likely source of funding—up to $300,000—described extensive prep work already completed by me and others, and requested only (1) feedback to finalize product design, (2) help adding treatment info for up to ten emergent causes of chest pain, (3) use by twenty-five to fifty members, and (4) help testing use effectiveness. I also explained how product use could be expanded over time as an adjunct to how members currently earn CME credits and prepare for board exams.

A few other board members expressed interest in the project during brief conversations and in other ways. A majority of members, however, rejected my submitted proposal (I wasn't invited to present it face-to-face). They did so without notifying me. I learned about it through that organization's executive director, who also provided no explanation.

Such Fear Prevented a Solution to ACO Dysfunction

Even Dr. Michael Hunt, who expressed a clear understanding of the IT needed to make ACOs more functional (chapter 5), wasn't willing or able to discuss the needed change called for in those IOM reports and other sources. He is no longer trying to help SVHP become an ACO.

Such Fear Ended a Series of Internet Healthcare Conferences

When I registered for an Internet Healthcare 2000 conference, the cochair responded: "Dear friend, I'm thrilled you'll be attending our conference. Please be my guest at a ($250) pre-event sit-down dinner." I was baffled. She didn't know me. At first, I assumed the event was bombing, but when I arrived, the place was packed. People were standing in the street because there was no more room inside. When I tracked her down, she explained, "I couldn't get doctors to come." At one point during the conference, there were only five physicians in an audience of several hundred attendees. The fact that doctors didn't attend and how problematic that was came up repeatedly from the podium and in private conversations. The following year that conference was only half as large. Two years later it was canceled because of physician nonattendance. Healthcare marketers and digital information vendors now attend a different annual healthcare internet conference,* but physician participation is minimal.

PHYSICIANS HAVE NO NEED TO FEAR CHANGE

When the US board certification process was established in 1933, physicians had no choice but to process all or most care info from memory only. In the 1970s, the TV show *Marcus Welby, M.D.* was popular, and US doctors were considered pillars of society and secular high priests who somehow spoke for God. All of that perpetuated the notion that doctors know everything they need to know. Perpetuating that image worked then, but today no doctor

---

*   HCIC website: https://www.hcic.net

can be expected to have complete mastery of all or most needed info via memory only. Trying to appear as if they do is no longer an effective way to preserve physician status and income.

- The information doctors need to process has grown exponentially, and demand for cost-effective care adds a whole new dimension.

- The people physicians interact with, especially in EDs, stopped buying into the notion of doctor omniscience a long time ago.

- Documenting and reporting competent, cost-effective care after processing related info, especially diagnostic, only from memory has become enormously burdensome.

Given the exponential growth of healthcare complexity and costs, mastering the use of the IT needed to process so much related info will be more than enough to justify physician status and incomes.

Doing so will also let physicians lead the way toward solving the biggest problems now plaguing healthcare, secure their rightful place at its center, and enjoy more respect, autonomy, and job satisfaction.

Finally, use of color-assisted, Bayesian-like analysis to generate EHR data needed to produce functional AI/ML products which they can fully interact with will keep doctors in the driver's seat for a very long time.

CHAPTER 8

What You Can Do to Propel Needed Change

> *The quickest, surest, and most direct way to initiate needed change is by persuading a US EM organization to do so.*

I say this for several reasons:

- At this point, physicians are likely the only people in the industry who can and will propel change.

- Burnout, the main reason for doing so, is most problematic among emergency physicians who can implement change as a professional organization.

- Use of better IT permitting color-assisted, Bayesian-like analysis is the key to addressing burnout.

- HIPUS, LLC is fully prepared to implement that technology.

- By collaborating with the ABEM, which administers certification exams, an EM professional organization could likely construct a comprehensive knowledge base in about five years—and a marketable knowledge base in fewer than two years.

- The aforementioned technology and knowledge base can be implemented and expanded over time without disrupting how ED physicians now earn CME credits, prepare for board exams, and interact with patients.

After this IT has been used to address ED physician burnout, it can be modified and expanded for use in that and other settings to further improve care quality and reduce costs. Also, after ED physicians accept the need for and use of such IT, other doctors will more likely do so.

> *Whether you live in the US or elsewhere, you can propel implementation of the HIPUS® system by requesting use of such IT in a letter addressed to the executive director of a US EM organization or in an email message sent to a general address provided by that organization. You can do so effectively as a doctor or nonphysician.*

In that letter or message, you might describe how you or someone you know has been adversely affected by physician burnout, uneven care quality, or out-of-control costs, and explain why you see use of the HIPUS® system as a solution to the problem. The excerpts of letters sent to Governor Rendell (chapter 7) provide examples of what you might say as a nonphysician. Such letters addressed to an EM organization will be much more effective.

There are actually three such organizations: the American College of Emergency Physicians (ACEP), the American Academy of Emergency Medicine (AAEM), and the American College of Osteopathic Emergency Physicians (ACOEP). While each is independent of the others, their members often work together to achieve shared objectives. Sending the same letter or email to all three will maximize its effectiveness. Contact information for each organization is provided at the end of this chapter.

> *You can propel needed change more effectively by urging others to read this book and respond in the same way. Word of mouth always has been, and remains, a powerful tool.*

If you're a physician who is or isn't burned out and you understand the need for such IT in order to solve the problem of burnout, you can likely prompt other doctors to read and respond to it in the same way—including burned-out ED physicians. Those doctors might, in turn, do the same.

If you're a nonphysician and you understand the need for such IT to address any of the problems described, you can likely persuade other nonphysicians to read and respond to it—people who might then do the same.

If you're a nonphysician professional working to improve healthcare management and/or policy, you might be especially well positioned to prompt others (nonphysicians *or* doctors) to read this book and respond to it.

If you're a doctor's significant other, family member, or friend and are directly affected by their burnout, you might be especially well positioned to prompt that doctor to read and respond to this book.

If you're a physician or nonphysician leader serving as an ACO executive, physician educator, med school dean, residency director, EHR vendor executive, or innovation center director, you will surely be well positioned to encourage doctors or nonphysicians to read and respond to it.

The ripple effect of such steps, taken by you and others, can persuade an EM organization to implement needed IT.

Buying this book and persuading others to do so will help that organization take the first step by implementing a study product.

Proceeds from book sales will be needed and used to do that. Assuming successful submission of an NIH SBIR grant proposal (chapter 7), proceeds from book sales will be needed to supplement the money provided by that program to implement *and test* a HIPUS® study product. The money provided (about $300,000) will be enough to complete both tasks, but the time allotted (one year) won't be. I and those who built the study product prototype will need money to do preparatory knowledge base and RDB work *after* we've been notified of the program's decision to provide grant money and *before* the money is actually provided and that allotted time period begins. The time distance between those events is usually about six months. Prep work done during that time period will be critical to successful completion of the aforementioned two tasks within a year.

If enough people buy this book, we can implement and test a study product much more quickly and efficiently by not having to apply for and use federal grant money.

Implementing that product successfully will pave the way for creation and use of bedside assistance. Doing so will help doctors understand the need for and prepare them to use bedside assistance. Physicians who understand the need can help persuade a hospital or healthcare system to implement it. Public or private funding needed to do so can be much more easily secured, and the 21st Century Cures Act can effectively counter US industry resistance. Successful implementation at one hospital or healthcare system can attract funding for and propel implementation elsewhere.

The EM organization contact info follows:

EM Professional Organization Contact Info

American College of Emergency Physicians
Executive Director: Sandy Schneider
Email address: sschneider@acep.org
Mailing address: ACEP, PO Box 619911, Dallas, TX 75261-9911

American Academy of Emergency Medicine
General email address: info@aaem.org
Executive Director: Tamara Wagester
Mailing address: 555 East Wells Street, Suite 1100, Milwaukee, WI 53202-3823

American College of Osteopathic Emergency Physicians
General email address: info@acoep.org
Executive Director: Amanda Mahan
Mailing address: ACOEP, PO Box 1488, Warrenville, IL 60555

ACKNOWLEDGMENTS

I WAS BLESSED to connect and collaborate with the following professionals who helped me secure patent protection for, and then prepare in other ways to implement, the HIPUS® system.

Steven J. Rocci—Steve, then a partner at Woodcock Washburn LLP in Philadelphia, helped me secure patent protection for use of colors to convey finding sensitivity and specificity. Because the patentability of doing so was a contested issue, I interviewed several attorneys before asking Steve to prepare a patent application. His work was flawless. His application sailed through the US and Canadian patent offices without a glitch. Also, because Steve understood that the measure of a patent is in its claims, he focused on producing the claims and let me focus on describing the invention. Over time, I came to greatly appreciate the value of those claims. Because of healthcare industry resistance to change, the patent expired before the invention could be implemented, but it prompted, and allowed me to fully design, the HIPUS® system independently. It can now be implemented much more easily and to much greater effect.

Andrew Goldman—After submitting the patent application, I collaborated with Speed Graphics in New York City to produce HIPUS®-related promotional material, including a multimedia presentation. Andrew helped me convert a fifty-one-page voice-over script to a much better seventeen-page script. The presentation he and Speed Graphics helped me produce elicited most of the healthcare pioneer responses described in chapter 6.

Roy Yokelson—"Uncle Roy," owner of Antland Productions in New York City and Emmy Award–winning sound designer and recording engineer, produced the voice-over and sound effects for the multimedia presentation. Roy went to extraordinary lengths to produce high-quality content. He recruited two of the best voice-over talents in the US, persuaded them to *reproduce* some content to perfect it, and insisted on reproducing all the voice-over I created. He also edited much of the latter at no additional charge. Working with Roy was a thoroughly delightful experience.

Joanna Schlesinger and Joe Chielli—Joanna and Joe, website designer and photographer at Church Street Studios in Philadelphia, helped me create the first HIPUS® website. Having no related experience, being a burned-out physician at the time, and wanting to largely replicate what Speed Graphics had created despite producing a very different product made me a difficult client. My demands made creating that website many times more difficult than it needed to be. Because I was in awe of the voice-over Roy Yokelson produced, I insisted on including it on the website. To permit use of the site by people who either didn't want or couldn't use audio, we essentially combined two sites into one—a hugely complicated and time-consuming task. Joanna and Joe gave me everything I asked for. Looking back, I'm amazed by how competently and graciously they performed that task.

Michael J. Hernandez—Michael's best-selling *Database Design for Mere Mortals* has earned worldwide respect by providing an effective way to learn RDB design. His book provides clear, easily understood, step-by-step instructions for designing a soundly structured database including tables, fields, keys, table relationships, business rules, and views. Using his book allowed me to design an RBD for use with HIPUS® study and bedside assistance applications—a task I never could have done otherwise. Mike also took the time to help me connect with Armen Stein, a premier database designer in Seattle, who prompted me to improve that RDB design in several ways.

Bill Denk—Bill, while at Open Professional Group, helped me design HIPUS® mobile bedside assistance for use by ED physicians when caring for patients. Bill demonstrated exceptional user interface expertise and an innate sense of how to create applications that people can easily understand and use. One of the applications he created was number two on a short list selected by Steve Jobs himself to launch the iPad. Bill also helped me switch from PC to Mac computer use and learn how to use Adobe Illustrator and Photoshop to design and illustrate bedside assistance. He also created the HIPUS® logo I now use.

Darius Samani—After earning a PhD in electrical and computer engineering and an MBA at the University of Texas at Austin, Dr. Samani founded VersaSuite, an EHR vendor. He and his team built a complete healthcare information system using one code set and database, which provides an intuitive, identical inpatient and outpatient user interface. Darius has expressed interest in and supported my efforts to implement the HIPUS® system for many years. He and his team are highly qualified to incorporate mobile bedside physician assistance into EHRs. He recently provided time and cost estimates of nine months and $500,000 for incorporating the assistance Bill and I designed into his preexisting EDIS. I now realize that he can incorporate any type of physician assistance into any EHR system.

Bob Bajoras and Daisey Traynham—Bob and Daisey, vice president and creative director at Art+Logic, a custom software, application, and website development firm, helped me produce demo prototypes illustrating use of the HIPUS® study and bedside assistance applications. They also created websites providing access to both. Recently, they and others at Art+Logic produced a detailed, step-by-step description of how the HIPUS® study product might be implemented, along with time and cost estimates for completing each step. Conversations with Art+Logic professionals about how each of the previously described steps might be performed revealed an abundance of related expertise. Bob and Daisey were an absolute joy to work with.

Ayoub Zekhnini and Myles Ingram—Ayoub and Myles, data scientists living in Morocco and New Jersey, helped me create applications that can use ICD-10 codes, extracted via a National Center for Health Statistics browser tool, and large sets of ED records to calculate the incidence of each corresponding disease as the primary cause of a particular ED chief complaint (e.g., chest pain). Doing so required close collaboration between all three of us. Ayoub and Myles did a superb job of creating and providing online access to those applications.

Myles also helped me produce chapter 3 of this book. Most importantly, he helped me understand the need for data quality to optimize AI/ML product performance—discussed in that chapter.

Matthias Gruber—Matthias, a data scientist living in Germany, helped me understand and use LLMs. He created the OpenAI API assistant described in chapter 3, which I used to update part of the HIPUS® knowledge base. He also helped me understand how an LLM might be used to update that entire knowledge base with much greater ease and speed.

Sheila Buff—Sheila is a highly experienced writer, ghostwriter, developmental editor, and book coach. She has written or contributed to the writing and publication of numerous books and other publications covering consumer-oriented medicine and health, including eight national bestsellers and numerous Amazon best sellers and top titles. As a book coach, her expertise, skills, and interest in the subject matter were tremendously helpful to me during the writing and publication of this book.

I connected with Sheila through Kevin Anderson & Associates in New York City, which provides book writing, editing, and publishing assistance. The team I worked with during the writing of this book and initial publication efforts were also immensely helpful.

Evan Schnittman, Tate Causey, and Elizabeth Brueggemann—Evan, Tate, and Elizabeth serve as Chief Publishing Officer, Authority Advisor, and Production Editor at Advantage Media Group, the exclusive book publisher for Forbes Media. They directed and coordinated all work related to the publication, promotion, sales, and distribution of my book—work performed by an extraordinary team of experienced and talented professionals. Their careful attention to, and regard for, my every expressed concern or request made collaborating with them immensely rewarding.

ABOUT THE AUTHOR

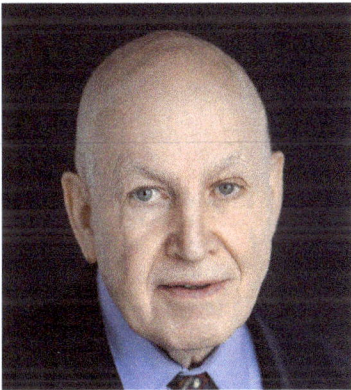

Mark Sorensen, MD

PHYSICIAN, INVENTOR, DESIGNER

After earning an MD at the University of Utah, I did three years of residency training at Tulane Medical Center—two years in surgery, one in internal medicine. During my education and training, I discovered a passion for diagnosis and a related aptitude for the practice of emergency medicine (EM).

I was an average med student in most ways but earned the highest score in the class on my physical diagnosis final.

During my surgical training, while we were rounding on patients at Charity Hospital in New Orleans, Earl Peacock, chairman and department of plastic surgery, said to us, "The practice of medicine consists of three things: diagnosis, diagnosis, and diagnosis." I didn't expect to hear that from a plastic surgeon, but realized it was true—especially in the practice of EM. Diagnosis constitutes the bulk of EM practice and permeates every part of it.

As a first-year surgical resident, I had to run the "Accident Room" (the surgical side of the emergency department [ED]) at Charity Hospital. At the time, it was one of twelve major trauma centers in the US. Before beginning that rotation, I seriously doubted I could do it and believed I might well be excluded from the program after an attempt. Instead, I discovered an aptitude for the job, which was the biggest surprise of my life. I found I could care for up to twenty patients at a time, to the satisfaction of four senior residents. I was later asked to repeat that rotation when a fellow resident wasn't able to perform the required tasks.

During my training, the realization that my being gay would never change precipitated an existential identity crisis, which derailed pursuit of a conventional career. Instead, I decided to work in EDs to earn a living and design a way to diagnose to my satisfaction. That decision determined the content of my life's work—locum tenens (as needed) ED work and, primarily, designing and preparing to implement better diagnostic assistance.

As preparation for both, I spent about two years studying the diagnosis of 150 causes of abdominal pain, thirty causes of chest pain, and twenty causes of headache. While doing so, I realized that using colors to convey the significance of the presence (specificity) or absence (sensitivity) of findings (symptoms, signs, and test results) in ruling in or out diseases let me learn, recall, and apply that info much more effectively and with greater ease and speed.

I later realized that linking all other care information—costs of and indications for tests, referrals, treatments, and hospitalizations—to diagnoses (diseases) or diagnostic assistance (findings) within a relational database is the best way to make it immediately available when needed.

The use of color-coded diagnostic data became the cornerstone of the HIPUS® system, which will let physicians fully process diagnostic data and fully integrate use of all care and patient data, while interacting with patients and making decisions. They can thereby improve care quality and reduce costs at every care point.

During each phase of the HIPUS® project, I did what I could myself and then collaborated with others who had the expertise needed to complete that phase. I love collaborating with others and was blessed to connect with people having abundant expertise and great capacity for collaboration. I and several of those collaborators are now prepared to implement the HIPUS® system.

ENDNOTES

1   Peckham C. Medscape Lifestyle Report 2017: Race and ethnicity, bias and burnout. Medscape. Published January 11, 2017. https://www.medscape.com/features/slideshow/lifestyle/2017/overview?faf=1

2   Kane L, et al. Physician burnout & depression report: Stress, anxiety, and anger. Medscape. Published January 21, 2022. https://www.medscape.com/slideshow/2022-lifestyle-burnout-6014664.

3   Shanafelt TD, Hasan O, Dyrbye LN, et al. Changes in burnout and satisfaction with work–life balance in physicians and the general US working population between 2011 and 2014. *Mayo Clin Proc.* 2015;90(12):1600-1613. doi:10.1016/j.mayocp.2015.08.023

4   Arora M, Asha S, Chinnappa J, Diwan AD. Review article: Burnout in emergency medicine physicians. *Emerg Med Australas.* 2013;25(6):491-495. doi:10.1111/1742-6723.12135

5   Stehman CR, Testo Z, Gershaw RS, Kellogg AR. Burnout, drop out, suicide: Physician loss in emergency medicine, Part I [published correction appears in *West J Emerg Med.* 2019 Aug 21;20(5):840-841]. *West J Emerg Med.* 2019;20(3):485-494. doi:10.5811/westjem.2019.4.40970

6   American Medical Association. What should be done about the physician burnout epidemic. Updated February 16, 2023. https://www.ama-assn.org/practice-management/physician-health/what-should-be-done-about-physician-burnout-epidemic

7   Kane L, et al. Physician burnout & depression report.

8   Institute of Medicine (US) Committee on Quality of Health Care in America. *To Err Is Human: Building a Safer Health System.* National Academies Press; 2000. doi:10.17226/9728

9   Institute of Medicine (US) Committee on Quality of Health Care in America. *Crossing the Quality Chasm: A New Health System for the 21st Century.* National Academies Press; 2001. doi:10.17226/10027

10   Institute of Medicine Committee on the Learning Health Care System in America. *Best Care at Lower Cost: The Path to Continuously Learning Health Care in America.* National Academies Press; 2013. doi:10.17226/13444

11   Peckham C. Medscape Lifestyle Report 2017.

12   Kane L, et al. Physician burnout & depression report.

13   Shanafelt TD, Hasan O, Dyrbye LN, et al. Changes in burnout and satisfaction with work–life balance in physicians and the general US working population between 2011 and 2014.

14   Arora M, Asha S, Chinnappa J, Diwan AD. Review article: Burnout in emergency medicine physicians.

15   Stehman CR, Testo Z, Gershaw RS, Kellogg AR. Burnout, drop out, suicide.

16   Kane L, et al. Physician burnout & depression report: Stress, anxiety, and anger.

17   Kane L, et al. Physician burnout & depression report.

18   Institute of Medicine (US) Committee on Quality of Health Care in America. *Crossing the Quality Chasm: A New Health System for the 21st Century.* National Academies Press; 2001. doi:10.17226/10027.

19   Emanuel EJ. Reforming American medical education.

20   Lucey CR, Davis JA, Green MM. We have no choice but to transform: the future of medical education after the COVID-19 pandemic. *Acad Med. 2022*;97(3S):S71-S81. doi:10.1097/ACM.0000000000004526.

21   Benbassat J. Changes in Medical Education.

22   Matathia S, Tello M. Medical education needs rethinking.

23   Mohta NS, Johnston SC. Medical education in need of a 2020 revamp.

24   Institute of Medicine (US) Committee on Quality of Health Care in America. *Crossing the Quality Chasm.*

25   Page L. Docs Struggle to keep up with the flood of new medical knowledge. Here's advice. Medscape. Published March 2, 2023. https://www.medscape.com/viewarticle/989043?form=fpf

26   Institute of Medicine (US) Committee on Quality of Health Care in America. *Crossing the Quality Chasm.*

27   Institute of Medicine Committee on Diagnostic Error in Health Care, and Board on Health Care Services. *Improving Diagnosis in Health Care.* National Academies Press; December 29, 2015. doi:10.17226/21794

28   Olson APJ, Graber ML. Improving diagnosis through education. https://pmc.ncbi.nlm.nih.gov/articles/PMC7382536/

29   Graber ML, Holmboe E, Stanley J et al. A call to action: next steps to advance diagnosis education in the health professions. Diagnosis (Berl). 2021 Dec 8;9(2):166-175. doi: 10.1515/dx-2021-0103.

30   Agency for Healthcare Research and Quality. Current state of diagnosis education. Last reviewed March 2022. https://www.ahrq.gov/diagnostic-safety/resources/issue-briefs/education-dx-outcomes-3.html

31   Olson APJ, Graber ML. Improving diagnosis through education.

32   Edlow JA, Pronovost PJ. Misdiagnosis in the emergency department: time for a system solution. *JAMA.* 2023;329(8):631-632. doi:10.1001/jama.2023.0577

33   Li MLJ, McNamara R, Newman N, Galer M, Secura A. *The Reclamation of Emergency Medicine: "Take EM Back" White Paper.* Take Medicine Back, PBLLC; July 12, 2021. https://takemedicine-back.org/site/assets/files/1070/reclamation_of_emergency_medicine_white_paper.pdf

34   Alexander L, Scheffler R. Study finds private equity investment accelerates concentration and

undermines a stable, competitive healthcare industry. American Antitrust Institute. Published May 18, 2021. https://www.antitrustinstitute.org/work-product/study-finds-private-equity-investment-accelerates-concentration-and-undermines-a-stable-competitive-healthcare-industry/

35 Li MLJ, McNamara R, Newman N, Galer M, Secura A. *The Reclamation of Emergency Medicine: "Take EM Back" White Paper*.

36 Li MLJ, McNamara R, Newman N, Galer M, Secura A. *The Reclamation of Emergency Medicine: "Take EM Back" White Paper*.

37 Kroth PJ, Morioka-Douglas N, Veres S, et al. Association of electronic health record design and use factors with clinician stress and burnout. *JAMA Netw Open*. 2019;2(8):e199609. doi:10.1001/jamanetworkopen.2019.96099

38 Sinsky C, Colligan L, Li L, et al. Allocation of physician time in ambulatory practice: a time and motion study in 4 specialties. *Ann Intern Med*. 2016;165(11):753-760. doi:10.7326/M16-0961

39 Hill RG Jr., Sears LM, Melanson SW. 4000 clicks: a productivity analysis of electronic medical records in a community hospital ED. *Am J Emerg Med*. 2013;31(11):1591-1594. doi:10.1016/j.ajem.2013.06.028

40 de Dombal FT, Leaper DJ, Staniland JR, McCann AP, Horrocks JC. Computer-aided diagnosis of acute abdominal pain. *Br Med J*. 1972;2(5804):9-13. doi:10.1136/bmj.2.5804.9

41 de Dombal FT, Leaper DJ, Horrocks JC, Staniland JR, McCann AP. Human and computer-aided diagnosis of abdominal pain: further report with emphasis on performance of clinicians. *Br Med J*. 1974;1(5904):376-380. doi:10.1136/bmj.1.5904.376

42 Dzulkifli MA, Mustafar MF. The influence of colour on memory performance: a review. *Malays J Med Sci*. 2013;20(2):3-9.

43 Institute of Medicine Committee on Diagnostic Error in Health Care, and Board on Health Care Services. *Improving Diagnosis in Health Care*. National Academies Press; December 29, 2015. doi:10.17226/21794.

44 Artificial intelligence and machine learning (AI/ML)-enabled medical devices. U.S. Food and Drug Administration. Updated Dec 6, 2023. https://www.fda.gov/medical-devices/software-medical-device-samd/artificial-intelligence-and-machine-learning-aiml-enabled-medical-devices

45   Berner ES, Webster GD, Shugerman AA, et al. Performance of four computer-based diagnostic systems. *N Engl J Med.* 1994;330(25):1795. doi: 10.1056/NEJM199406233302506

46   Berner ES, Webster GD, Shugerman AA, et al. Performance of four computer-based diagnostic systems.

47   Rotmensch M, Halpern Y, Tlimat A, Horng S, Sontag D. Learning a health knowledge graph from electronic medical records. *Sci Rep.* 2017;7(1):5994. doi:10.1038/s41598-017-05778-z

48   Chen IY, Agrawal M, Horng S, Sontag D. Robustly extracting medical knowledge from EHRs: a case study of learning a health knowledge graph. *Pac Symp Biocomput.* 2020;25:19-30.

49   Mohammed S, Budach L, Feuerpfeil M, et al. The effects of data quality on machine learning performance on tabular data. *arXiv preprint arXiv:2207.14529.* Published 2022. https://arxiv.org/pdf/2207.14529

50   Sehgal R. AI needs data more than data needs AI. Forbes. Published October 5, 2023. https://www.forbes.com/sites/forbestechcouncil/2023/10/05/ai-needs-data-more-than-data-needs-ai/#:~:text=All%20aspects%20of%20AI—machine,%22training%20fuel%22%20for%20AI

51   Data quality metrics & measures: what you need to know. Informatica. https://www.informatica.com/resources/articles/data-quality-metrics-and-measures.html#:~:text=Common%20data%20quality%20metrics%20include,%2C%20validity%2C%20duplication%20and%20uniqueness

52   Mohammed S, Budach L, Feuerpfeil M, et al. The effects of data quality on machine learning performance on tabular data.

53   Baum D. *Generative AI and LLMs for Dummies.* Snowflake Special Edition. John Wiley & Sons, Inc.; 2024.

54   Institute of Medicine Committee on Diagnostic Error in Health Care, and Board on Health Care Services. *Improving Diagnosis in Health Care.*

55   Gleason K, Harkless G, Stanley J, Olson APJ, Graber ML. The critical need for nursing education to address the diagnostic process. *Nurs Outlook.* 2021;69(3):362-369. doi:10.1016/j.outlook.2020.12.005

56   Institute of Medicine Committee on Diagnostic Error in Health Care, and Board on Health Care Services. *Improving Diagnosis in Health Care.*

57   Institute of Medicine (US) Committee on Quality of Health Care in America. *To Err Is Human: Building a Safer Health System.*

58   Institute of Medicine (US) Committee on Quality of Health Care in America. *Crossing the Quality Chasm.*

59   Institute of Medicine Committee on the Learning Health Care System in America. *Best Care at Lower Cost.*

60   Institute of Medicine (US) Committee on Quality of Health Care in America. *To Err Is Human: Building a Safer Health System.*

61   Institute of Medicine (US) Committee on Quality of Health Care in America. *Crossing the Quality Chasm.*

62   Institute of Medicine Committee on the Learning Health Care System in America. *Best Care at Lower Cost.*

63   Bates DW, Singh H. Two decades since *To Err Is Human*: an assessment of progress and emerging priorities in patient safety. *Health Aff (Millwood).* 2018;37(11):1736-1743. doi:10.1377/hlthaff.2018.0738

64   Dzau VJ, Shine KI. Two decades since *To Err Is Human*: progress, but still a "chasm." *JAMA.* 2020;324(24):2489-2490. doi:10.1001/jama.2020.23151

65   Bates DW, Singh H. Two decades since *To Err Is Human*: an assessment of progress and emerging priorities in patient safety.

66   Dzau VJ, Shine KI. Two decades since *To Err Is Human*: progress, but still a "chasm."

67   Institute of Medicine (US) Committee on Quality of Health Care in America. *Crossing the Quality Chasm.*

68   Institute of Medicine (US) Committee on Quality of Health Care in America. *Crossing the Quality Chasm.*

69 Connor L, Dean J, McNett M, et al. Evidence-based practice improves patient outcomes and healthcare system return on investment: findings from a scoping review. *Worldviews Evid Based Nurs.* 2023;20(1):6-15. doi:10.1111/wvn.12621

70 Institute of Medicine (US) Committee on Quality of Health Care in America. *Crossing the Quality Chasm.*

71 Institute of Medicine Committee on the Learning Health Care System in America. *Best Care at Lower Cost.*

72 Hixon T. The U.S. does not have a debt problem … it has a health care cost problem. Forbes. Published February 9, 2012. https://www.forbes.com/sites/toddhixon/2012/02/09/the-u-s-does-not-have-a-debt-problem-it-has-a-health-care-cost-problem/?sh=75b9a2f46eb7

73 Government's mandatory health care spending now exceeds entire discretionary budget. U.S. House Budget Committee. Published January 26, 2024. https://budget.house.gov/press-release/governments-mandatory-health-care-spending-now-exceeds-entire-discretionary-budget#:~:text=In%202024%2C%20federal%20spending%20on,to%20skyrocket%20to%20%243.103%20trillion

74 Hanson M. Average cost of medical school. Education Data Initiative. Last updated November 9, 2024. Accessed January 16, 2024. https://educationdata.org/average-cost-of-medical-school

75 Hardy A. Health insurance and medical costs are set to surge again in 2024. Money. Published January 12, 2024. https://money.com/health-insurance-premiums-increase-2024/

76 Lopes L, Montero A, Presiado M, Hamel L. Americans' Challenges with Health Care Costs. KFF. Published March 1, 2024. https://www.kff.org/health-costs/issue-brief/americans-challenges-with-health-care-costs/

77 Kendall D. Millions of Americans are struggling with medical debt. Governing. Published April 10, 2024. https://www.governing.com/finance/millions-of-americans-are-struggling-with-medical-debt#:~:text=Medical%20debt%20affects%20100%20million,declare%20bankruptcy%20at%20age%2025

78 Hoffman DP, Mertzlufft J, Taylor R. Chronic disease prevention 2024 update: essential to our health and future. *Annals of Bioethics & Clinical Applications.* 2024;7(1). doi:10.23880/abca-16000269

79   Cutler D. The world's costliest health care … and what America might do about it. *Harvard Magazine.* May-June 2020. https://www.harvardmagazine.com/2020/04/feature-forum-costliest-health-care

80   Why are Americans paying more for healthcare? Peter G. Peterson Foundation. Last updated January 3, 2024. https://www.pgpf.org/blog/2024/01/why-are-americans-paying-more-for-healthcare

81   Institute of Medicine Committee on the Learning Health Care System in America. *Best Care at Lower Cost.*

82   Medicare Shared Savings Program Continues to Deliver Meaningful Savings and High-Quality Health Care. CMS press release, published on October 29, 2024. https://www.cms.gov/newsroom/press-releases/medicare-shared-savings-program-continues-deliver-meaningful-savings-and-high-quality-health-care

83   Shared Savings Program Fast Facts – As of January 1, 2025. https://www.cms.gov/files/document/2025-shared-savings-program-fast-facts.pdf

84   Medicare ACO participation flat in 2022: NAACOS issues a call to action for CMS to spur ACO growth. NAACOS. Published January 26, 2022. https://www.naacos.com/press-release--medicare-aco-participation-flat-in-2022#:~:text=NAACOS%20Issues%20a%20Call%20to,increased%20to%20483%20in%202022

85   Casalino LP, Gans D, Weber R, et al. US Physician Practices Spend More Than $15.4 Billion Annually to Report Quality Measures. Health Aff (Millwood). 2016 Mar;35(3):401-6. doi: 10.1377/hlthaff.2015.1258

86   Saraswathula A, Merck SJ, Bai G, et al. The volume and cost of quality metric reporting. *JAMA.* 2023;329(21):1840-1847. doi:10.1001/jama.2023.7271

87   Institute of Medicine (US) Committee on Quality of Health Care in America. *Crossing the Quality Chasm.*

88   Gillespie G. ACO complexity, lack of IT maturity is burning out MDs. Health Data Management. Published March 8, 2016. https://www.healthdatamanagement.com/articles/aco-complexity-lack-of-it-maturity-is-burning-out-mds

89   Weil TP. Why are ACOs doomed for failure? *J Med Pract Manage.* 2012;27(5):263-7. PMID: 22594055.

90   Bernstein DN, Crowe JR. Price transparency in United States' health care: a narrative policy review of the current state and way forward. *Inquiry*. 2024;61. doi:10.1177/00469580241255823

91   Fair Health Consumer. Your Costs. https://www.fairhealthconsumer.org/#answer2

92   Institute of Medicine (US) Committee on Quality of Health Care in America. *Crossing the Quality Chasm*.

www.ingramcontent.com/pod-product-compliance
Lightning Source LLC
Chambersburg PA
CBHW040143200326
41519CB00032B/7586